Yoga
for
Runners

Christine Felstead

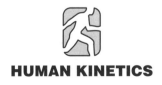

HUMAN KINETICS

Library of Congress Cataloging-in-Publication Data

Felstead, Christine.
  Yoga for runners / Christine Felstead.
    pages cm
1. Running--Training. 2. Yoga. I. Title.
  GV1061.5.F46 2013
  181'.45--dc23

                            2013012604

ISBN-10: 1-4504-3417-7 (print)
ISBN-13: 978-1-4504-3417-1 (print)

This publication is written and published to provide accurate and authoritative information relevant to the subject matter presented. It is published and sold with the understanding that the author and publisher are not engaged in rendering legal, medical, or other professional services by reason of their authorship or publication of this work. If medical or other expert assistance is required, the services of a competent professional person should be sought.

The web addresses cited in this text were current as of July 2013 unless otherwise noted.

Acquisitions Editor: Diana Vincer; **Developmental Editor:** Anne Cole; **Assistant Editor:** Tyler Wolpert; **Copyeditor:** Patsy Fortney; **Permissions Manager:** Martha Gullo; **Graphic Designer:** Joe Buck; **Graphic Artist:** Tara Welsch; **Cover Designer:** Keith Blomberg; **Photograph (cover):** © eyetrigger Pty Ltd/Corbis RF/age fotostock; **Photographs (interior):** Tim Bermingham/© Human Kinetics; **Photo Asset Manager:** Laura Fitch; **Visual Production Assistant:** Joyce Brumfield; **Photo Production Manager:** Jason Allen; **Art Manager:** Kelly Hendren; **Associate Art Manager:** Alan L. Wilborn; **Illustrations:** © Human Kinetics, unless otherwise noted; **Printer:** United Graphics

We thank Mindful Body Works in Toronto, Ontario, for assistance in providing the location for the photo shoot for this book.

Human Kinetics books are available at special discounts for bulk purchase. Special editions or book excerpts can also be created to specification. For details, contact the Special Sales Manager at Human Kinetics.

Printed in the United States of America   10 9 8 7 6 5 4 3 2

The paper in this book is certified under a sustainable forestry program.

Human Kinetics
Website: www.HumanKinetics.com

United States: Human Kinetics
P.O. Box 5076
Champaign, IL 61825-5076
800-747-4457
e-mail: humank@hkusa.com

Canada: Human Kinetics
475 Devonshire Road Unit 100
Windsor, ON N8Y 2L5
800-465-7301 (in Canada only)
e-mail: info@hkcanada.com

Europe: Human Kinetics
107 Bradford Road
Stanningley
Leeds LS28 6AT, United Kingdom
+44 (0) 113 255 5665
e-mail: hk@hkeurope.com

Australia: Human Kinetics
57A Price Avenue
Lower Mitcham, South Australia 5062
08 8372 0999
e-mail: info@hkaustralia.com

New Zealand: Human Kinetics
P.O. Box 80
Torrens Park, South Australia 5062
0800 222 062
e-mail: info@hknewzealand.com

E5765

I dedicate this book to that global community bonded by a love of running. May it inspire you to marry your passion for running with the practice of yoga and maintain an openness to the potential of your mind, body, and spirit to produce the outcomes you seek.

Christine Felstead

Contents

Pose and
Sequence Finder

Pose	Full description on page	Used in sequence(s) on page(s)
Ab curls I	111	199, 219
Ab curls II	112	199, 219
Boat	120	207
Bound angle	162	186, 196, 207, 214
Bound side stretch	153	205, 212
Bridge	121	189, 197, 207, 218
Cat–dog stretch	87	188, 219
Chair forward bend	235	NA
Chair hip stretch	239	NA
Chair staff pose	231	NA
Chaturanga (yoga push-up)	114	199, 200, 203
Chest opener	94	203, 220, 225
Child's pose	88	188, 204, 219, 220, 225
Cobra	95	192, 220, 225
Cow pose, shoulder stretch	123	186, 196, 226
Deep breathing	242	NA
Desk downward dog	233	NA
Dolphin (downward dog variation)	116	201, 225
Dolphin plank	117	201, 225
Double pigeon	160	196, 207, 214
Downward dog	89	188, 189, 192, 193, 194, 200, 201, 202, 203, 204, 206, 210, 211, 212, 213, 216, 218, 220, 222, 223, 224, 225, 226
Downward dog (leg extended variation)	151	203, 209
Eagle arms	124	224
Ear to shoulder	122	226

Pose	Full description on page	Used in sequence(s) on page(s)
Equal standing	61	192, 194, 195, 196, 199, 200, 204, 205, 206, 212, 216, 217, 222, 223, 224
Equal standing, arms overhead	84	187, 192, 199, 224
Extended side stretch	152	195, 205, 223
Finding the gluteus maximus	145	209
Gate	137	193, 216
Half downward dog	86	187, 220
Half frog	73	203, 217, 222
Hamstrings curl	131	214
Hamstrings eccentric stretch	130	214, 223
Hero pose	64	186, 192, 222
Hero toes	65	186, 192
Internal rotator stretch	163	214
Knee to ankle balance	157	187, 206
Kneeling clam	149	209
Kneeling quadriceps stretch	170	211
Legs up the wall	182	221
Lizard	167	203, 211
Locust	96	204, 217, 220
Lunges (low, kneeling, and high)	164	189, 193, 194, 201, 202, 203, 210, 211, 212, 216, 222
Lunge twist	166	193, 194, 202
Pigeon	159	189, 194, 206, 213
Plank	113	192, 199, 200, 203
Plantar massage	62	186, 221
Quadriceps and iliotibial band rollouts	74	186, 221
Relieve eye strain	241	NA
Revolved triangle	135	195, 205, 216
Savasana (corpse pose)	97	189, 197, 208, 214, 218, 221, 223, 226
Seated chair twist	234	NA
Seated forward bend	138	206, 218
Seated wide-leg forward bend	139	207, 218
Side plank	115	200

(continued)

Poses *(continued)*

Pose	Full description on page	Used in sequence(s) on page(s)
Simple balance	63	195
Simple chest stretch	236	NA
Simple seated twist	91	196, 207, 220
Squat	161	187, 196
Staff pose	90	196, 206, 213, 218, 220, 226
Standing Egyptian	155	205, 212
Standing forward bend	132	192, 199, 204, 222, 224
Standing side bend	85	187, 224
Standing wide-leg forward bend	136	188, 217
Straight-leg lunge	134	195, 216
Supine hamstrings stretch	140	197, 207, 218
Supine twist	93	189, 208, 221, 226
Supported bound angle	178	NA
Supported bridge	179	NA
Supported chest opener	177	NA
Supported child's pose	181	NA
Supported forward bend	180	NA
Tabletop with leg extended	150	209
Tabletop wrist stretch	240	NA
Thighs to chest	92	189, 197, 207, 214, 218, 221, 223
Toe spreading	66	186
Tree	158	196
Triangle	133	204, 217
Twisted lizard	168	203, 211
Upward dog	119	199, 200, 225
Upward plank	118	207, 226
Wall squat	72	222
Warrior II	154	195, 205, 223
Warrior III	156	205, 216

Essential Sequences

Sequence title	Description	Duration	Page
Sequence 1: TV yoga	Poses to do during leisure time	As long as desired	186
Sequence 2: no excuses post-run	An easy sequence that you can do with running shoes on	5-8 minutes	187
Sequence 3: runners' hot spots	Short post-run tune-up	10-15 minutes	188
Sequence 4: weekly overall tune-up	Overall body balance practice that's great for active recovery	60-75 minutes	190
Sequence 5: strength and stamina	A challenging sequence to build strength and flexibility	75-90 minutes	197

Body Part–Specific Sequences

Sequence title	Description	Duration	Page
Sequence 6: hips	Increases range of motion and strengthens the hips	45-60 minutes	209
Sequence 7: hamstrings	Lengthens and strengthens the hamstrings	45-60 minutes	214
Sequence 8: back	Increases flexibility and strength and eases lower-back pain	45-60 minutes	219
Sequence 9: knees	Decompresses, strengthens, and balances the knee joint	30-40 minutes	221
Sequence 10: upper body	Eases shoulder and neck tension	30-40 minutes	224

While it is tempting to jump right into a yoga practice, investing some time to prepare and understand the poses is recommended. The asanas are described in detail, including valuable alignment details, positioning tips, anatomical focus, and related benefits, in chapters 6-11. It is important to read these details, even if you are familiar with the pose—there may be a new aspect to experience. Chapter 12 contains the sequences, which use a variety of poses for a desired focus. The sequences provide instructions for transitioning from one pose to the next, holding times, and any related details. You should be familiar with the pose alignments and easily able to perform each pose before you begin the sequences. If you are starting yoga to promote recovery from an injury, be sure to read chapter 14, as you may need to modify some of the poses described in the sequences. Remember alignment, breath, and mindfulness pave the way for a safe and sustainable yoga practice.

Introduction

Runners love to run—and so they should! Running is a fabulous sport that invigorates the body and mind. There is nothing more inspiring than seeing a runner's long, rhythmic stride, observing the look of determination and focus, and sensing the feelings of euphoria and freedom that come with every step. Unfortunately, most runners experience some form of injury during their running careers. This, of course, causes much stress and discontent and may explain the propensity to try to run through injuries. *Yoga for Runners* is a comprehensive program that helps keep runners healthy and doing the sport they love.

There is no such thing as being too stiff to do yoga; in fact, the stiffest have the most to gain. Yoga is a personal practice and, unlike running, requires no quantifying. It is simply a catalyst to help the body return to a level of balance and symmetry. Yoga gives every body exactly what it needs. For some, flexibility is the biggest gain, whereas for others, the strengthening component is more important. And every runner will gain tremendous benefit from yoga breathing and meditation.

EFFECTS OF RUNNING

Recognizing running's growing popularity among millions worldwide, let's take a look at its physical impact.

The average runner strikes the ground 1,000 times per mile, 50 to 70 times per minute per foot, with a force of two to three times their body weight. Although the foot is the initial point of contact, the impact is felt throughout the body. Depending on the efficiency of the running stride, running affects, to some degree, all of the muscles, tendons, ligaments, and bone structures of the body. Therefore, it isn't a surprise that the majority of runners sustain some form of running-related injury during their careers.

To varying degrees, running affects these parts of the body:

- Feet
- Ankles
- Shins
- Calves
- Quadriceps
- Iliopsoas
- Hamstrings
- Pelvis
- Hip joints
- Spine
- Elbows
- Shoulders
- Neck

Running is a repetitive sport, meaning that the same groups of muscles are used repetitively. All movement, such as walking and running, requires muscles to work in a coordinated fashion through a series of contractions and extensions. When muscles are contracted repeatedly, their fibers shorten and, over time, remain in the shortened state. This phenomenon is not unique to running; rather, it is simply the way the human body works—use the same muscles repeatedly, and the constant contractions will result in their overall shortening. Any athletic movement or static holding pattern in the body produces this effect. For example, a common modern-day injury as a result of computers and handheld devices is carpal tunnel syndrome, a repetitive strain injury most commonly associated with holding the hands and wrists in certain positions for extended periods of time.

As muscles shorten, they create imbalances in the musculoskeletal system and reduce the range of motion in related joints. Many runners' injuries are a direct result of some form of musculoskeletal imbalance related to repetitive movement. For example, tight outer quadriceps and weak inner quadriceps create an imbalance in the knee joint, which can manifest as knee pain and lead to runner's knee.

COMPOUNDING EFFECTS OF SITTING

All runners have been warned of the ill effects of running. Running injuries are certainly a factor, but clearly the benefits outweigh the risks. However, it is important to understand that running alone cannot be blamed for many runners' afflictions. Running exacerbates conditions that already exist in the body as a result of other things we do—particularly, sitting for prolonged periods of time.

Sitting is the number one position in the workplace today, and it is typically done with less than perfect posture. The human spine was not designed to be sat on for the number of hours many of us do, and this is a major cause of lower-back pain and neck and shoulder tension. The shape that the body assumes for hours on end for days and years eventually becomes the shape it assumes at all times. The older we are, the more time we have spent sitting and the more ingrained these patterns are in our bodies.

The following sections describe the effects on the body as a result of sitting for prolonged periods.

Lower Back   Most of us sit with less than perfect posture, often slouching in our chairs. This puts considerable stress on the lumbar spine, compressing the lumbar vertebrae and tightening the erector spinae muscles that support the spine.

Core Strength   When we sit for prolonged periods in chairs, our bodies become accustomed to having chairs supporting our weight rather than engaging our core muscles. Conversely, sitting or standing in a proper, posturally aligned upright position engages the abdominal and back muscles to support the torso.

Shoulders and Upper Back   When a person is seated at a computer, at a desk, or in a car, the upper back is often rounded, with the shoulders raised and the chest caved in. This affects overall spinal alignment and tightening of the neck and shoulder muscles. Many people suffer from persistent tightness and tension in the shoulders and neck, leading to chronic discomfort, pain, and even headaches.

Hips   While in a seated position, the hip joints are locked at 90 degrees and the external rotator muscles tighten and shorten. Over time, the ability to externally rotate the femur is diminished and the range of motion in the hip joint is reduced. Tightness in the hips can lead to overall pain and discomfort in the hip region and also affects the lower back and knees. Additionally, the hip flexors, including the quadriceps and the iliopsoas muscles, are contracted while in a seated position, which further affects posture and contributes to lower-back problems.

Hamstrings   The hamstrings are inactive and held in a shortened state in the seated position, contributing to their overall tightening. Considering that many of us have been sitting for hours a day since grade school, it is easy to understand the compounding effect this has on the hamstrings. Tight hamstrings also contribute to lower-back tightness and pain.

Yoga is an ancient health system that has surged in popularity in recent years. The physical practice of yoga involves postures, or asanas, that stretch, strengthen, and tone the muscles, allowing the musculoskeletal system to regain balance and symmetry. On a subtle, yet profound, level, yoga works on the energetic body. Through yogic breathing, you can access the subtle, yet powerful, energetic body and mind. The myriad of annoying aches and pains will start to ease and eventually disappear with a consistent yoga practice that is targeted to your specific needs. Let this book become a companion to guide you to a more holistic state of fitness. Not only will you be able to carry your body through daily activities with greater ease, comfort, and confidence, but you will also add longevity to your sport as you become a healthier and more balanced runner.

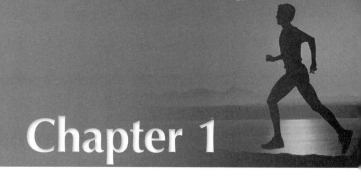

Chapter 1

A Fit Body

Being fit enables us to go through daily life with physical ease and be free of chronic aches and pains. Being fit also improves our quality of life, providing the strength and stamina to keep up with active children and perform household chores and other daily tasks with little effort or difficulty. Being fit provides energy to put toward both work and play.

Health includes a number of measurable values (e.g., blood pressure and cholesterol levels) and encompasses being free from sickness and disease. It also includes mental health and is supported with good nutritional choices. A fitness regimen should contribute to an overall healthy state of physical and mental well-being.

WHY DO WE RUN?

Running is one of the most popular ways to maintain fitness. There are a reported 36 million runners in the United States and an additional 40 million fitness walkers, and the numbers are growing annually, according to RunningUSA.org. The classic and most popular races sell out in record times, and to fill the demand there is an unprecedented growth in the number and variety of road races, including various distances and those for specialized sectors of the population.

There are good reasons that running is so popular. Namely, it is relatively inexpensive, almost everyone can do it, it can be done anywhere, and it brings tremendous health benefits. According to Running USA's National Runner Survey, people run for the following reasons:

- To stay in shape (75.5 percent women; 75.2 percent men)
- To stay healthy (74.8 percent women; 70.8 percent men)

- To relieve stress (62.4 percent women)
- For fun (58.9 percent men)
- For exercise (25.3 percent women; 22.0 percent men)
- Because they competed in school and never stopped (15.2 percent men)
- Due to weight concerns (13.8 percent women)

BENEFITS OF RUNNING

As you can see, staying in shape and staying healthy are two of the major reasons people run, and they're directly related to some of the sport's major benefits. Let's take a look at these benefits in more detail.

Manages Weight   Running is one of the most efficient forms of exercise to maintain an ideal body weight. Running is a rigorous form of exercise, burning an average of 100 calories per mile. So, running 5 miles a day can burn 500 calories in a relatively short time. Although many runners are drawn to running for weight loss, they remain motivated to keep weight off.

Improves Cardiovascular Health   Running is good for the heart, making it stronger and more efficient. Running can lower blood pressure and help arteries maintain their elasticity. Running improves blood circulation and raises HDL (high-density lipoprotein, the "good" cholesterol). A healthy cardiovascular system can reduce the risk of heart attack and stroke. So, while running improves your outward appearance, it also improves the overall functioning of your body.

Improves Bone Health   The physical demands of running help retain muscle mass, and bones respond by becoming stronger. To maintain strong and healthy bones, especially as we age, exercise is vital. Weight-bearing activity, which requires the muscles to work against gravity, is particularly beneficial. This includes exercises that are done while standing, such as running, and exercises that use either the person's body weight (yoga) or equipment (weights) to work the muscles. Actions that require muscles and bones to carry weight helps them become stronger. Along with a healthy diet, this can reduce the risk of osteoporosis.

Manages Stress   Many people today are plagued by stress, and running is a great way to manage its ill effects. Whether providing time to think about life problems or to escape them for a while, running releases tension as the miles fly by. Often, problems that appeared unsolvable subside after a run. Stress often leads to insomnia, and a regular running routine can improve the ability to sleep and rest.

Improves Psychological Health Running can alter mood as a result of the release of endorphins. These hormones create a sense of euphoria, often referred to as a "runner's high," and can result in overall mood enhancement. According to Michael Sachs and Gary Buffone in *Running as Therapy: An Integrated Approach*, running is often used to treat clinical depression and other psychological disorders. Some doctors claim that running works as well as psychotherapy in helping patients with clinical depression. Running makes patients less tense, less depressed, less fatigued, and less confused.

Increases Self-Esteem From a young age we are conditioned to achieve goals, and who doesn't like the feeling of accomplishment and pride that ensues? For a runner, entering his first race and crossing the finish line can create a tremendous sense of triumph that ultimately boosts self-esteem and confidence. Short races become longer races, marathons turn into ultramarathons, and race times decrease as we achieve new personal bests—and each new feat is accompanied by an increased sense of self-satisfaction.

Allows Social Interaction In spite of the well-known cliché "the loneliness of the distance runner," running can be a very social sport. This is particularly the case today with running clinics, clubs, teams, and corporate events. Many lasting friendships result from becoming running buddies, and running events and training runs often extend into other social functions. The various channels of social media have created new ways for runners to share their passion with no geographic boundaries. An entire social network has developed around running, from websites where runners can meet other runners to blogs where runners share their experiences.

Is Simple to Do In spite of all of the high-tech running gear sold in many stores, running is a very simple sport. Almost everyone can run in any location with little to no gear. With just a good pair of running shoes and a sidewalk, beach, or park trail, a runner is set to explore—no membership or expensive equipment is necessary.

With all of these benefits, it's no wonder the sport is experiencing unparalleled growth and that runners become addicted to running!

A HEALTHY BODY

Unquestionably, running offers tremendous health benefits, but some aspects of the sport frustrate the runner's objectives and produce unfavorable results in the body. As detailed in the introduction, most notably running creates stiffness and muscular imbalances that can cause pain, discomfort, and injury. However, while running may exacerbate conditions in the body, it is not the sole culprit.

For example, consider posture as it relates to running. Every runner knows the importance of good running form to create an efficient stride. The upper body needs to be relaxed, the hips and hamstrings need to have enough range of motion to permit fluid motion, and the core muscles need to be strong enough to support the torso while in motion.

However, our posture is the most deeply rooted habit in our bodies, and the postural tendencies adopted during the day carry over into our running posture. Furthermore, running exacerbates many of the ill effects of sitting all day. Chiefly, the hips, which are locked at 90 degrees while seated, will only tighten further during a run, as will the hamstrings. The lower back, which is compressed while seated, will compress further with the added weight-bearing impact of running.

Recall that one of the main reasons people run is to be healthy. A healthy body is injury—and, for the most part, pain free. A healthy and fit body moves easily, has energy for life's adventures, and has the strength to meet life's physical demands. With this definition in mind, are these the characteristics of a fit person?

- Easily running 26 miles but having difficulty bending over to tie one's shoelaces
- Waking up stiff and in some degree of pain every morning
- Walking with a limp
- Ignoring chronic pain

Of course not! A person in tune with her body and wishing to stay healthy can read the warning signs of trouble, and recognize when to lower training intensity. Healthy muscles should be balanced in flexibility and strength, supporting the skeletal system and not pulling bone structures out of alignment. Healthy muscles and joints should facilitate movement rather than impede it, and healthy joints should maintain a reasonable degree of their intended range of motion.

Therefore, in this book, a healthy and fit body will be defined as a balance of the following:

- Flexibility
- Endurance
- Strength
- Cardiorespiratory endurance

Yoga for Runners defines fitness from a perspective of overall health and balance and presents a program designed to eliminate many of the daily aches and pains. *Yoga for Runners* restores the body to balance and symmetry, liberating it from the extreme tightness that restricts movement and consumes energy. When the body returns to a state of greater balance, many of the nagging aches and pains that we learn to live with, or simply attribute to aging, diminish and eventually cease. It is in this state that the body is truly healthy and fit. It is also in this state that risk of injury is reduced and we can keep running!

REFERENCES

Sachs, M. and G. Buffone. 1997. *Running as Therapy: An Integrated Approach.* Northvale, N.J.: Jason Aronson.

Chapter 2

The Running–Yoga Connection

How does a 5,000-year-old Eastern spiritual practice become the hot trend of the Western world? Clearly, people are drawn to yoga for a number of reasons, but what keeps them coming back is how they feel after the practice. The desire to move away from high-impact aerobics, the interest in more holistic and healing forms of exercise, and the aging population likely have contributed to the growing interest in yoga. As yoga has become more mainstream, it has made its way into amateur and professional sport organizations, corporate boardrooms, schools, and penitentiaries, just to name a few venues. In this chapter we examine specifically why runners need yoga.

WHAT IS YOGA?

Prior to yoga becoming mainstream in Western society, the typical image of a yogi was someone from the East with a long beard sitting in a full lotus position in a transcendent meditative state with incense burning close by. Today, the image is more likely to be a model sporting fashionable yoga clothing that accentuates every contour of her perfectly toned body. The promise of a yoga body is used to promote DVDs, books, diets, and magazines. So it is no wonder that, for many, yoga is perceived as another form of exercise.

Exercise involves a form of physical activity in which the body moves with some degree of intensity to raise the heart rate and work the muscles. The goal of exercise is to achieve a level of physical fitness. Although the forms of exercise are endless, they all meet this basic definition, and the focus is primarily on the physical.

Using the words *exercise* and *yoga* in the same sentence is disdainful to some yoga gurus; nevertheless, there is no doubt that the physical aspect of yoga is what draws many people to the practice. Additionally, physical postures (asanas) are just one of the eight limbs (structural framework) of yoga practice. Furthermore, all definitions of yoga include an aspect of mind and body. The following definitions of yoga, taken from well-known yoga texts, all include an aspect of the physical body—but with more complexity and depth than simply the exercise component.

> The word yoga is derived from the Sanskrit root yuj meaning to bind, join, attach and yoke, to direct and concentrate one's attention on, to use and apply. . . . [It is] the yoking of all the powers of body, mind and soul . . . .
>
> B.K.S. Iyengar, *Light on Yoga*

> Yoga means union. The union of the individual soul with the Universal Spirit is yoga. Yoga is the union of the body with the mind and of mind with the body.
>
> B.K.S. Iyengar, *The Tree of Yoga*

> One [interpretation of the word yoga] is "to come together," "to unite." . . . Another meaning . . . is "to tie the strands of the mind together."
>
> T.K.V. Desikachar, *The Heart of Yoga*

People are drawn to yoga for reasons that are as personal and varied as the individuals themselves. Some are curious to see what all the fuss is about, others desire to be more flexible, whereas still others seek to calm the mind or learn to meditate. Regardless of the intent, after a yoga class people typically feel good—physically stretched out, taller, released of physical tension, mentally calmer, and more relaxed. On a deeper level than happens with other forms of exercise, the body and the mind have united, which the mind registers as a positive experience.

EFFECTS OF YOGA ON RUNNERS

Runners are often reluctant to try yoga; their most common fear is that they are not flexible enough. It is not uncommon for those attending their first *Yoga for Runners* class to ask whether the room will be filled with lithe and flexible bodies, in spite of the class being advertised "For runners; no yoga experience necessary." This fear may be driven by the many media images showing people in advanced yoga poses, fueling the notion that you have to be able to bend like a pretzel to do yoga. This is the furthest thing from the truth. Yoga is suitable for every body type. It can be started at any age regardless of physical condition, and those who are the stiffest have the most to gain. Runners, specifically, have a tremendous amount to gain from adding yoga to their fitness regimens.

Running can lead to injury because of its repetitive nature and the resulting musculoskeletal imbalances. On a physical level, yoga restores balance and symmetry to the body, making it the perfect complement to running. Runners are often drawn to yoga to deal with specific issues, such as improving flexibility or helping with an injury. Yet many are shocked at the world it opens for them, specifically, the strengthening capacity and the use of muscles they never knew they had. Let's take a closer look at the effects of yoga, both physical and mental, on runners.

Physical Effects

As seen in the preceding definitions, yoga encompasses more than the mere physical postures. Nonetheless, the physicality of yoga is what draws most people to their first yoga class. The following summarizes the physical benefits that runners can expect from yoga.

Flexibility   Many runners cite greater flexibility as the number one reason for beginning a yoga practice. This is a good reason, because yoga stretches the muscles that are tight, which in turn increases the range of motion in related joints. Increased flexibility decreases stiffness, results in greater ease of movement, and reduces many nagging aches and pains.

Strength   Runners are strong in ways that relate to running. However, a running stride involves only the lower body and movement in one plane—sagittal (i.e., forward and backward). Thus, certain muscles become strong while others are underused and remain weak. Runners have strong legs for running, but when faced with holding a standing yoga pose, they are quite surprised to find that their legs feel like jelly. This is simply because a properly aligned yoga pose involves using all the muscles in a variety of planes. The muscles that are weak fatigue quickly, and those that are tight scream for release—thus, the jelly-leg syndrome.

Overly tight muscles are also weak ones. To be fully functional, a muscle needs to contract when needed and also relax and lengthen when needed. For example, if your hand is perpetually in a state of contraction, as in a fist, its function is severely impaired. A healthy muscle is able to move through a healthy range of motion.

Additionally, running primarily uses the muscles from the hips down, whereas a balanced yoga practice involves the entire body. Muscles that are simply not used while running are called upon and strengthened—specifically in the arms, upper torso, abdominals, and back. Moreover, yoga uses the person's own body weight to create resistance, working against gravity to build the muscle and bone strength vital for overall health. Muscles strengthen by various methods of contraction, followed by rest and supported with proper nutrition. In running, the strengthening is primarily in the legs, whereas a balanced yoga practice contracts and stretches the muscles of the entire body. For example, a fairly basic pose such as plank requires numerous muscles to actively engage; otherwise, the effect of gravity would result in the belly, hips, and upper torso sagging.

Strengthening the upper body and core helps improve posture during daily activities and also while running. Moreover, a strong core allows the arms and legs to move more efficiently, creating better overall form, less fatigue, less weight impact on the legs, and a reduced risk of injury. A strong core creates a strong runner!

Additionally, a by-product of becoming stronger is greater muscle tone. Yoga helps shape long, lean muscles that do not hinder free range of movement in joints.

Biomechanical Balance Overusing some muscles while underusing others creates muscular imbalances, which affect the entire musculoskeletal balance and impairs biomechanical efficiency. For runners, biomechanical imbalances eventually lead to pain and injury.

Depending on the action, a muscle is either contracting (i.e., an agonist) or lengthening (i.e., an antagonist). For example, if you make a fist and lift your forearm, the biceps contracts while the triceps stretches. If you want showy biceps and do repeated biceps curls to pump up the muscle, the triceps will shorten and you could lose the ability to straighten your arm.

A healthy balance is to work to both contract and stretch to maintain muscle equilibrium as well as functionality. For example, when stretching the hamstrings, the quadriceps need to contract. This coordinated action not only creates a deeper and safer hamstring stretch, but also provides an opportunity to strengthen the quadriceps, especially the inner quadriceps, which are weak in many runners. This is crucial for runners because the hamstrings most likely need lengthening while the commonly weak inner quads need strengthening.

Executed correctly, a seemingly simple yoga pose requires the balanced activity of opposing muscle groups. To hold a pose, some muscles need to stretch while others need to contract. In this way, a natural balancing of strength and flexibility occurs, which creates biomechanical balance over time. This is one of the major benefits that await runners who undertake a regular yoga practice.

Every yoga pose is a balance of stability (muscles contracting and strengthening) and mobility (muscles stretching and lengthening). At no time is only one muscle group used. Even the simplest yoga pose requires an awakening of every part of the body. Downward dog (chapter 7) is an exemplary pose to demonstrate this. Following is a summary of the major muscle actions in this fundamental pose.

Stability (Strength)

- Arms: hands, wrists, lower arms, triceps, deltoids
- Back: lower trapezius, serratus anterior
- Legs: quadriceps, tibialis anterior (front of shins)

Mobility (Flexibility)

- Arms: fingers, biceps
- Back: latissimus dorsi, paraspinals (both superficial and deep layers of back muscles)
- Legs: hamstrings, calves, Achilles tendon

A balanced yoga practice requires most of the muscles in the body to perform some action. At the same time, joints are taken through their full ranges of motion as the corresponding muscles contract or stretch to support the movement. The result is improved muscle balance, which translates to better form, stronger running, and fewer injuries.

A Complete, Inside-Out Body Workout   Yoga provides a workout that includes every muscle and all the joints. Yoga uses all muscle groups, including the small muscles in the hands and toes, the large muscles of the legs and torso, the superficial muscles such as the calves and hamstrings, and the deeply layered muscles that are not visible. When examining a person in the downward dog pose, you can see clearly that the superficial muscles of the back are stretching. What is less obvious is the lengthening of the intrinsic layer of paraspinal muscles, creating space and decompressing the vertebrae.

Furthermore, all of the body's systems beyond the muscle groups are worked in yoga, including the cardiovascular, respiratory, skeletal, and endocrine systems. Additionally, the internal organs are massaged and oxygenated through yogic breathing and movement in the poses.

An Energized Body   Many forms of exercise deplete the body of its energy stores. Yet a yoga practice oxygenates the blood and creates more energy, leaving the body and mind feeling restored and energized. Yoga provides a vehicle through which the body can actively recover from the physical demands of running.

Improved Breathing   Lung capacity is of prime importance for runners, because it creates the ability to maintain an even breathing pattern through all phases of running. The better the lung capacity is, the more oxygen is circulated through the system, which is most helpful for running long and strong. However, the breathing pattern used in running and other forms of aerobic exercise involves quick and shallow inhalations and exhalations. This uses only the top portion of the lungs, leaving the middle and lower portions untouched. Yogic breathing involves slow, deep inhalations and long exhalations, making use of the upper, middle, and lower portions of the lungs. Yogic breathing has been shown to increase lung capacity, and greater lung capacity increases endurance and improves overall athletic performance.

In Sanskrit, *prana* means "energy," and yogic breathing is called *pranayama* (see chapter 3 for more detail). Through the breath, you bring in oxygen, feeding your cells and creating vital life force, and remove carbon dioxide, eliminating toxins. The use of the breath in yoga is vital. Whereas holding the breath creates internal tightness, tension, and anxiety, deep breathing releases tension, reduces stress and anxiety, and physically helps the body ease into poses, particularly those that are challenging. Through this conscious breathing, the body is energized as a result of increased oxygen circulation throughout all of its systems.

Mental Effects

Recall that the preceding definitions of yoga all share an aspect of uniting body and mind. Through concentrating on the yoga pose and uniting it with the breath, the mind remains unified with the body, which improves both physical and mental well-being. Following is a summary of the mental effects of yoga.

Mind–Body The effects of running have significant parallels to the meditative aspects of yoga. Yoga practice teaches you to stay in tune with your body and connected to the breath. Running, especially longer distances, requires this same discipline. It is easy to see that the awareness that yoga develops will enhance your ability to remain focused, calm, and in tune with your body during challenging runs. After all, running can be meditation in motion!

Body Awareness As a runner, you understand your body in relation to running. Yoga demands awareness of the entire body, from head to toe (including gross movements of dynamic yoga poses and subtle movements used in breathing) and large to small muscles. As yoga students quickly discover, no part of the body is untouched by yoga. As your awareness increases through yoga, you will be able to control smaller movements of your body or even feel the movement inside your body while simply being still. This increased awareness of your body in a yoga practice will translate into being more in tune with your body while running. The subtler signals that your body gives can lead to more enjoyable running and even injury prevention.

Calmness   A monkey mind is one that jumps from thought to thought—like a monkey jumping from tree to tree. The monkey mind is not content with simply being in the present moment, but rather, jumps about, typically moving backward or forward in time. Yoga asana practice is physically demanding and requires mindful concentration in the body. This brings a sense of calmness to the mind. Yoga classes typically include at least a few moments of sitting quietly and simply breathing. The simple act of sitting and observing the breath while eliminating the stream of thoughts that otherwise permeate our mind is the foundation of meditation. Meditation is known to produce a state of relaxation and a tranquil mind. The mind control practiced on the yoga mat can transfer to calmness and ease in running.

Stress Reduction   All forms of physical activity are good for relieving stress, and this is particularly true of yoga. The practice provides a much-needed break from the source of stress. Concentrating on the movement and the breath seems to melt away the daily issues that cause stress. A yoga practice provides the mental clarity to put things into better perspective, and problems often diminish in intensity. On a physiological level, yoga stimulates the parasympathetic nervous system (the branch of the nervous system involved with healing and the nourishment of the body), allowing the body and mind to heal while relieving the pressures related to the fight-or-flight mode.

Mindful Eating   Yoga is a health system that encompasses far more than physical movement and breathing. Patanjali's *Yoga Sutras* is one of the revered texts on yoga philosophy and is considered a bible in the practice, providing yogis guidelines for life. Volumes of translations have been written on these topics, and because of yoga's current popularity, many more interpretations have been added in recent years. The *Yoga Sutras* form the basis of yoga's comprehensive and balanced philosophical ideals.

The yamas and niyamas described in the *Yoga Sutras* relate to universal morals and personal observances, and many of these can be applied to food. For example, the first yama is *ahimsa*, or nonharming, which raises the notion that what we eat should not be harmful to us or to other beings. This forms the basis for many yogis' vegetarian or vegan food choices. A further example is the first niyama, *shaucha*, or cleanliness of body and mind, which challenges us to think about the purity of our food, eliminating toxicity in our bodies and in our environment, and the effect of foods on our minds and emotions.

It is not uncommon for yoga practitioners to make diet changes. This can be driven by the greater awareness instilled by the yoga philosophy, along with an overall heightened awareness of internal and external body functions. On a mere physical basis, yoga is a detoxifying practice, and as your body becomes cleaner, many unhealthy cravings may dissipate and be replaced with the desire to eat whole and healthier foods. Furthermore, because of the strong mind–body connection during a yoga practice, you may become more mindful of the effects your food choices have on your body and mind.

The benefits that yogis attempt to achieve through these dietary adjustments would also benefit runners. There is no doubt that cleaner eating (the reduction of junk food, animal fats, and processed foods, along with the intake of more whole foods) improves health, which only compounds the positive effects of running. Additionally, this is a wholesome and healthy approach if you are interested in weight loss.

BENEFITS OF YOGA FOR RUNNERS

Yoga restores the body's balance and symmetry through the physical postures, especially sequences that are designed specifically for runners. Many runners experience tremendous benefits even after just one yoga class, often expressing that they feel taller, their lower backs feel better, and they have greater body awareness during runs and daily activities. Following a yoga class that focuses deeply on the hips and hamstrings, many runners are surprised at the greater fluidity and ease they feel in their stride the next time they go for a run.

Many benefits await the casual, avid, or competitive runner that will translate directly to improved and sustained running. Runners love to run, and yoga is the perfect companion to keep them healthy and on the road. Integrating some aspect of yoga into a daily and weekly routine will result in the following benefits.

Better Running One of the biggest benefits of yoga for runners is better running. As mentioned earlier, yoga stretches and lengthens muscles so they become more supple and able to react during a run. This decreases muscle stiffness and increases range of motion in joints—namely, the hips, shoulders, ankles, and spine. Specifically, longer hamstrings and less restricted hip joint mobility create a longer and more fluid running stride. In addition, the strength and length gained by the muscles help to stabilize the skeleton, resulting in faster running.

A flexible joint requires less energy to move through a wider range of motion, and a flexible body creates more energy-efficient movements. This results in greater ease while moving about throughout the day and potentially an improvement in athletic performance. Runs become less exhausting and more enjoyable.

Finally, balancing the sympathetic and parasympathetic nervous systems creates a more relaxed state in the body while running. When you are relaxed, your aerobic capacity is enhanced with the flow of more oxygen-rich blood through your body (see chapter 3 for greater detail).

Healing and Avoiding Injuries Improved symmetry, alignment, and balance through yoga prevent new injuries from occurring while healing stubborn, chronic, and recurring injuries. Yoga postures help align the knee joint while strengthening the arches of the feet for better shock absorption. This reduces the weight-bearing impact of running. Improved range of motion may also slow the degeneration of the joints, giving runners longevity in the sport they love.

Runners have a high threshold for pain and learn to live with many nagging aches and pains as part of daily living. They are often amazed at how many of these nagging discomforts are eliminated with a yoga practice. For example, nagging and chronic lower-back pain is often eliminated as increased flexibility in the hamstrings, hip flexors, and muscles that attach to the pelvis relieves stress on the lumbar spine (lower back).

Post-Race Recovery A yoga practice after racing helps to eliminate the stiffness caused by lactic acid buildup in muscle tissue. Runners who attend a yoga class the day after a marathon are often amazed at the speed of their recovery; they are able to go up and down the stairs without pain and stiffness in short order. With reduced recovery times, runners can get back on the road quickly and in good health.

Following are general comments made by runners after a few weeks of yoga:

- I feel lighter on my feet.
- I am more aware of my posture and shoulders while running.
- I am more aware of my daily posture and how I sit at my computer.
- I am more in tune with my breathing.
- I feel stronger.
- I feel more relaxed.
- I sleep better.
- I have fewer aches and pains.

Recall that one of the prime reasons for running is to enhance health. The numerous physical and mental benefits of yoga help to broaden and round out the one-dimensional aspect of running. Furthermore, with the high risk of injury related to running, practicing yoga helps runners remain healthy and maintain their running routine, and actually improves their running.

YOGA AS CROSS-TRAINING

Runners who become injured experience a high rate of frustration, and they count the days until they can get back on the road. They typically turn to some form of cross-training such as cycling or swimming. These alternate activities let the injured muscles rest, allowing the acute pain to subside. Depending on their nature, injuries often return once running resumes. This indicates that the original source of the injury has not been dealt with.

Cross-training is a great way to use various muscle groups and vary the stress placed on specific muscles. It can also reduce the risk of injury from repetitive strain or overuse. Yoga is an excellent cross-training method because it helps offset the negative impact of running. Rather than merely resting the muscles, yoga works to restore the body to better alignment, symmetry, and balance. As the body moves in this direction, the physical strain creating the injury in the first place diminishes, and over time, the injury subsides. The results are different for everyone because the factors vary by individual.

Many runners are motivated to give yoga a try when they are injured in the hope that it will be a silver bullet and instantly improve their condition, but this is an unrealistic expectation. A properly balanced yoga practice performed with regularity and patience works over time. Integrating yoga into a weekly routine ensures the cross-training effects over the long term. Moreover, yoga is an excellent way to actively recover from the physical demands of running, fueling the body for the next run so you are not physically fatigued and trying to run on empty.

Although there are no guarantees in life, a regular yoga practice is a safe bet for reducing the risk of injury or curing a current one. Many runners today are experiencing tremendous benefits, and the best results are from those who have made yoga part of their weekly workout routine. After some time they marvel at how injury free they have remained, regardless of the distance they run.

REFERENCES

Desikachar, T.K.V. 1995. *The Heart of Yoga*. Rochester, VT: Inner Traditions International.
Iyengar, B.K.S. 1966. *Light on Yoga*. New York: Schocken Books.
Iyengar, B.K.S. 1988. *The Tree of Yoga*. Boston: Shambhala Publications Inc.

Chapter 3

Breathing

Breathing is life! From your first moment to your last on this earth, you breathe. Breathing is one of the most basic autonomic responses in your body; that is, it occurs automatically without your direction. As a baby, you breathed very naturally—in a relaxed manner when you were calm, and rigidly gasping for air when you were in need of attention. Watching babies sleep is very instructive: Their bellies expand with the inhalation and relax with the exhalation. This way of breathing is called natural, or abdominal, breathing and creates a comfortable and relaxed state. Abdominal breathing is slow, effortless, and quiet. Breathing this way makes use of both the upper and lower portions of the lungs, expands the intercostal muscles between the ribs, and uses the diaphragm, a key muscle in the breathing process.

When you left childhood behind and learned to deal with the stresses of everyday life, your breathing patterns changed. You left behind relaxed abdominal breathing and replaced it with shallow chest breathing, using only the top portion of the lungs with no movement through the lower ribs, belly and diaphragm. Shallow breathing deprives the body of vital oxygen, and lack of oxygen can lead to low energy levels, muscle stiffness, and even heart disease. In contrast to the effects of deep breathing, shallow breathing creates tension in the upper body, neck, jaw, and face.

As an aerobic endurance sport, running increases lung capacity—especially during intense and demanding training. However, aerobic breathing involves a quick and shallow breathing pattern, inhaling and exhaling through the mouth. Mindfully and consciously expanding and controlling the breath through yogic breathing is an excellent way to enhance aerobic capacity. However, slowing down the breath and mindfully breathing fully and deeply is often a challenge for runners. There is tremendous benefit to be gained by runners integrating some deep yogic breathing with the physical yoga practice or solely as a breathing exercise. Deep, diaphragmatic breathing expands lung capacity, and breath control yields great benefits for both stamina and endurance, providing the edge to run faster with less fatigue.

YOGIC BREATHING

The practice of breathing in yoga is called *pranayama*. In Sanskrit, *prana* is vital energy, or life force and *ayam* is to extend, or control. The yogic sages had a profound understanding of the importance of the breath, and thus pranayama is one of the eight limbs of yoga. While pranayama can be performed independently, it is also fundamental to the physical practice of yoga as it strengthens the connection between the body and mind.

The methods of deep, yogic breathing should be used solely as breathing exercises and to accompany your physical yoga practice, not while running. During the aerobic demands of running, you will breathe through the mouth with shorter breaths. The benefits of practicing yogic breathing will naturally result in greater lung capacity and greater awareness of the breath. which will improve your running performance.

Although runners may not initially be drawn to yoga to improve their breathing, many are surprised at the deep effects of yogic breathing. The deep breathing that accompanies the physical aspects of yoga is what creates that feeling of calm that those new to yoga marvel at. There are unquestionable advantages for athletes who learn yogic breathing techniques: It can both improve running and help them better deal with the stresses of daily life.

Effects of Yogic Breathing on Runners

To be clear, we define yogic breathing as a full exhalation that empties the lungs from top to bottom, and a deep inhalation that fills the lungs from bottom to top. Yogic breathing techniques and their effects on health and longevity are constantly being examined and researched. Moreover, because the links between stress and disease are now well understood, yogic breathing is often offered as a method of stress reduction.

Two important elements of yogic breathing are the impact on the affected muscle groups and the diaphragm. Yogic breathing uses two major muscles groups, the diaphragm and the intercostals between the ribs. The gentle movement of these muscles during breathing helps to keep them supple and elastic. Not using these muscles, as in shallow chest breathing, causes them to become immobile, rigid, and weak. Abdominal yogic breathing also relaxes and softens the belly, an area where perpetual tension is often held.

Yogic breathing takes in more oxygen and releases more carbon dioxide than normal breathing. Because there are more blood capillaries in the lower part of the lungs, more oxygen is circulated and more carbon dioxide is expelled with each breath. In this way, yogic breathing strengthens the lungs and diaphragm, leading to greater cardiovascular efficiency.

On an inhalation, the lungs expand and the diaphragm moves downward as it contracts, and on an exhalation, the lungs contract and the diaphragm expands as it moves upward. These movements cause the diaphragm to massage the internal organs and rejuvenate them with new, oxygenated blood. The lymphatic system, which plays a major role in our immune system, also relies on muscular movement to collect and rid the body of toxins. Therefore, these movements also improve lymphatic circulation, boost immunity, and help detoxify the body.

Following are some additional effects of yogic breathing on runners:

- Releases chronic tension in neck and shoulders
- Reduces stress, muscular tension, anxiety, and even fear
- Releases endorphins, which can help relieve stress related aches and pains (headaches, insomnia, and backaches).
- Lowers blood pressure
- Improves breathing and overall symptoms in those with asthma or other pulmonary problems
- Improves oxygenation of the blood cells, a vital component in cellular structure and metabolic health
- Improves blood flow throughout the body and creates more energy
- Helps to clear and focus the mind
- Aids sleep

Benefits of Yogic Breathing for Runners

In addition to improving runners' overall health, yogic breathing offers tremendous running-related benefits. Whereas aerobic exercise increases aerobic capacity, yogic breathing further enhances and increases lung capacity. Mindful breathing techniques using both the upper and lower portions of the lungs improve cardiorespiratory performance by pumping oxygen-rich blood more efficiently to blood vessels. This sets the stage to expand the cardiorespiratory boundaries to improve athletic performance.

Learning to breathe deeply and mindfully improves your overall awareness of your breathing during your workout. Staying in tune with your breath helps you maintain an even and controlled breath while running and prevents overexertion of the lungs. Greater efficiency in breathing delivers more oxygen to your muscles so they remain more relaxed. Muscle cramps subside, and your body works more efficiently with less fatigue.

As detailed in chapter 1, posture and spinal alignment become compromised due to the number of hours many of us spend seated in front of computers. Poor posture, with the chest collapsed and the upper back rounded, becomes ingrained in muscle memory. This reduces the body's efficiency and the lungs' ability to fully expand. Improving posture results in holding the upper body more upright; the shoulders move away from the ears, and the chest opens. This simple improvement in posture creates more internal space so the lungs can be unencumbered, making it easier to breathe deeply. This improved posture eventually becomes ingrained when standing, sitting, and running.

Furthermore, yogic breathing helps balance the autonomic nervous system. The central nervous system unconsciously regulates our internal systems and has two branches: the sympathetic and parasympathetic nervous systems. The sympathetic nervous system induces a fight-or-flight response, responding to situations by releasing adrenaline; raising the heart rate and blood pressure; decreasing blood flow to the liver, bladder, and kidneys; and increasing blood flow to the muscles (temporarily providing greater muscular strength). The adrenaline rush feels good for a time but leaves you fatigued as your energy is used up and your body is left depleted.

The parasympathetic nervous system is involved with healing and nourishment of the body. It slows the heart rate and the breath; stimulates the digestive organs to absorb food and store energy; and stimulates the immune system. It allows us to easily move into rest and sleep deeply. It promotes cellular growth and regeneration, which are critical for good health.

By its very nature, running stimulates the sympathetic nervous system. Whether engaged to hunt food or escape from enemies, running is a direct fight-or-flight response. Fast- paced and stressful living further stimulates the sympathetic nervous system. For overall health and well-being the sympathetic and parasympathetic nervous systems need to be in balance. In a state of balance, a person is able to respond to challenges quickly and easily, yet be able to rest and be calm when the defensive mechanism is not needed.

Yogic breathing is one of a number of ways to stimulate the parasympathetic nervous system. Thus, as yoga works to restore the physical body to greater balance and symmetry, the central nervous system achieves greater balance as well.

Life is stressful at times, and how you manage stress determines your overall state of health. Although running is a tremendous way to manage stress, yoga and its companion, yogic breathing, provide another avenue for improving your overall fitness and health. Achieving a more balanced central nervous system will serve you well; you will be able to respond quickly when needed and slow down to promote healing at other times.

Ka Po's Story

I first became interested in yoga after learning about the physical benefits that many runners and athletes gain in their strength, flexibility, and balance. I had been recovering from a strained left adductor muscle (inner groin muscle), so my primary concern was injury prevention through working out muscle imbalances, and staying injury free through my first half-marathon training. After several weeks of yoga practice, I completed an 8K race and was pleasantly surprised by the lack of soreness in my adductor muscles and the quick post-race recovery time. Yoga quickly became a practice not only of necessity but of intelligence. I understood that yoga will allow me to run better, longer, and stronger.

Another benefit that I had not considered before I started my yoga practice was the impact on the quality of my breathing. Learning to take deeper and fuller breaths, particularly in poses that engaged muscles that were stiff, has seamlessly made way into my daily life and running. I first noticed a change in my breathing technique in everyday living situations when I found myself taking long, deep breaths during my daily commute on the train. I also found my breathing more controlled and at ease in my running. This is particularly the case when I do hill training, because doing nine hill repeats can be a physical and mental toll on the body. I often remind myself to stay on the breath and observe it. As long as my breathing is controlled and relaxed, the rest will take care of itself.

Yogic Breathing Basics

Pranayama involves numerous breathing techniques that modify the inhale–exhale ratio, breath retention, and belly pumping actions, which should be practiced under the guidance of a qualified instructor. However, the two breathing techniques described here are safe and simple to execute.

Yogic breathing, both the inhale and exhale, is done through the nose. As a runner, you will be accustomed to breathing through your mouth, so this may feel awkward at the start. It is always helpful to start a breathing session and a physical yoga practice session with a few minutes dedicated to simply observing the breath. The breath is what connects the internal body and mind with the outside world. Your breathing pattern on any given day, or even time of day, will be varied. Through simple observation, you will notice that your breathing pattern varies according to your mood; the inhalation or exhalation may feel smoother or more labored compared to the other; one side of the respiratory system may expand more than the other. After a few moments of paying close attention to your breath, it will respond by becoming slower, more even, rhythmic, and calmer,

While breathing, focus on the breath and try to keep your mind from wandering. Thoughts will enter your mind; watch them without judgment, but do not let them take root and they will disappear. The intention is to keep your attention on the breath—otherwise known as mindful breathing.

Abdominal Breathing

Abdominal breathing is an extremely valuable tool to have at your dispense when your mind is dwelling on negative thoughts; you are feeling stressed out, angry, or anxious; or you're having difficulty falling asleep. It is also a helpful technique to practice for a few minutes prior to a race, when nerves and jitters may be mounting.

Most of us are in a perpetual state of holding and sucking the belly in. This creates movement in the upper chest but no movement in the belly while breathing. As the name implies, abdominal breathing requires the belly to move while in a relaxed state (as babies do). On the inhalation, the belly expands and moves outward, and on the exhalation, the belly softens as it relaxes and draws inward. Abdominal breathing requires movement in the diaphragm, abdominals, and intercostals to create a full, deep, and natural breath.

Ujjayi Breathing

Ujjayi is a breathing technique that literally translates to "victorious breath" or "powerful breath" (the *u* refers to the upward flow of energy, and *jaya* means "victory"). Because this breathing technique produces a distinct sound, it is also commonly known as "breath with sound." Ujjayi breathing allows you to control the inflow and outflow of breath and increases the intake of oxygen. Unlike abdominal breathing, ujjayi breathing keeps the abdominals engaged, increasing pressure in the abdominal cavity to support the spine, which is why it is the companion breathing technique to be used during your physical yoga practice. You can also do it when you're feeling tired or lethargic for an energetic boost.

Ujjayi breathing involves consciously narrowing the passageway at the back of the throat, allowing you to control the inflow and outflow of breath. The slight closure, or narrowing, is produced by slightly constricting the air passageway at the back of the throat. The physical action is similar to that of blowing air on glasses when cleaning them. Anatomically, this involves half-closing the glottis, a piece of cartilage at the top of the voice box. As air travels through the larynx and over the vocal cords, a unique aspirant sound is created.

Listen to the sound produced during the inhale and exhale and make the breath and sound as even and smooth as possible. Although constricted, the back of the throat remains soft. The breath should not feel forced; nor should the sound have any aggression or be so loud that it can be heard across the room. The sound created is soft and pleasant and can become a focus of meditation.

BREATHING EXERCISES

Although you might think that breathing should be natural, learning deep yogic breathing technique takes time and practice. It is important to let go of expectation and judgment and simply enjoy the experience. At the beginning you may feel that the breath is not very deep, but with time, practice, and conscious work, it will naturally increase in volume.

Because breathing is an automatic response that you take for granted, the notion of setting yourself up "just to breathe" may be foreign. However, think of this as an exercise and as such, how and where you set up to do it is important.

For a more relaxing experience, or if this work is new to you, it may be easiest to start lying down. You can use a bolster (a large rectangular cushion commonly used in yoga practice) if you have one, or you can make one by folding a blanket so it is about 3 inches (7.6 cm) thick, 5 inches (12.7 cm) wide, and 30 inches (76 cm) long. Fold a second blanket in a smaller square to create a pillow.

Sit on the floor in front of the setup and lie back so the bolster (or folded blanket) supports your spine from the lumbar region to your skull and the small pillow rests at the base of your head. Your head should be higher than your heart, and your chin should be tilted slightly downward. Straighten your legs; however, if you have any pain in your lower back, bend them and keep your knees together and your feet hip-distance apart. Pull your shoulder blades down your back so your upper arm bones drape over the bolster (or folded blanket), and let your arms rest by your sides. See figure 3.1.

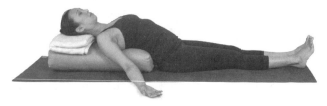

▶ **Figure 3.1**   Lying setup.

This setup supports your spine and opens your chest, which eliminates the stress of weight on your spine and facilitates deep breathing. Most people simply melt with comfort in this effortless setup, so if it isn't relaxing, move things about until it feels effortless.

Breathing exercises can also be done while seated. If you choose this method, it is best to sit on a surface to create some height (a folded blanket will work). Sit upright in a simple cross-legged position, ensure that both sitting bones are evenly grounded, lift your breastbone, and roll your arm bones back and your shoulder blades down to create the similar open chest position you achieved by lying over the bolster (or folded blanket). Pull your ribs and belly in to support your back, and let your chin drop slightly while lengthening the back of your neck. Relax your inner thighs. See figure 3.2.

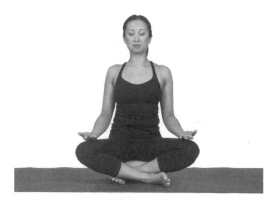

▶ **Figure 3.2**   Seated setup.

Once you are set up in your seated or lying position, these key points will guide you through your breathing exercise. Either breathing technique can be done, depending on your goal. If you want to de-stress, induce calm and rest, do the abdominal breathing technique. If you are preparing for a physical yoga practice or want to energize, do ujjayi breathing. Either method can safely be done at any time—the important thing is to practice deep, diaphragmatic breathing.

Observe: The first step when practicing a breathing technique is simply to observe your natural tendencies. For the first few minutes, lie comfortably on your setup and let your body and mind be still. Become aware of your breath and simply observe. How deep are you breathing? Is your breath smooth or harsh? Is there movement in your rib cage or belly? Is the movement even on the right and left sides of your body? Are the inhale and the exhale even? Does one feel easier? Observe the qualities of your breath without interference and without judgment.

Practice abdominal breathing: As you let go of being in a state of holding and sucking in your belly, let it completely relax. Place your hands on your lower belly, below your navel. Inhale and exhale through your nose. As you inhale, feel your belly expand into your hands, and as you exhale, feel it retract. Repeat this action and try to expand your belly a little more and let it fall to a relaxed state on the exhale. Do not push your belly up. Rather, allow it to simply respond to the slow and rhythmic filling and emptying of lungs with a relaxed belly. Practice this breathing technique alone at any time or as described above or for a few rounds prior to starting your ujjayi breathing.

Practice ujjayi breathing: Place the palms of your hands on the sides of your torso, letting your fingertips softly touch in the middle. Engage your abdominals by drawing in the navel and contracting the space between your two front hip bones, your pubic bone, and your navel. Constrict the back of your throat to start producing the ujjayi aspirant sound. As you inhale, feel your rib cage expand beneath your hands and your fingertips move apart. As you exhale, feel your rib cage contract and your fingertips touch.

Guide the breath: Begin to shape your breath to make it smoother and more regular. Gradually guide your breath from its naturally tendency toward a smoother and more even rhythm. Extend the exhale so that your lungs empty completely, from top to bottom, and on the inhale, let your rib cage expand as your lungs fill from bottom to top. Let the aspirant sound of the breath be your guide.

Try to make the length, effort, and feel of the inhale the same as that of the exhale to create a seamless flow of breath.

Give yourself time: At first, give yourself 10 to 15 minutes with this breathing exercise. Choose a space where there will be no disruptions. No disruptions means no cell phones, no television or radio, no music, no kids, no cats, no dogs—basically, try to eliminate anything that can cause a distraction. At first this may seem like a long time, but with practice, you will likely want to remain longer.

Select a time of day: The time of day to do a breathing practice is entirely up to you. First thing in the morning is a good time to remove the cobwebs and hone the mind. Before bed is very effective to eliminate the stresses of the day and get your body and mind ready for sleep; during the day is a good time to destress and energize the body and mind. Keep in mind that this breathing can be done any time, any place. Try it to reenergize when you are feeling tired, when you are stuck in traffic, when you are fighting to meet that deadline—whenever you find yourself in a stressful situation!

Go inside: When movement occurs in the outer body, there is corresponding movement on the inside as well. With every inhale, the diaphragm contracts to make space for the lungs to expand and receive the breath; with every exhale, the diaphragm expands, helping the lungs to empty. With this apparent stillness there is undulating movement throughout the body, energizing and calming at the same time. This way of breathing is also referred to as diaphragmatic breathing. Be mindful of the tendency to fill only the upper portion of your lungs and stopping when your upper chest expands. Train yourself to feel the lower portion of your rib cage expand. This brings air to the dark corners of the lungs where, through habit, the breath may be a little reluctant to penetrate. The mind and focus alone will open those spaces to receive a full and deep breath.

Like other aspects of yoga, ujjayi or abdominal breathing techniques may not come naturally; it has to be practiced with patience and focus. The effort has tremendous payback for both your running and daily life. As you become accustomed to deep breathing, you can use it as a tool whenever needed. In yoga practice you are constantly reminded to return your focus to your breath, so when facing a challenge in your run—say, at the bottom of a big hill—switch your focus to your breath and you will be at the top before you know it. As you anxiously await the sound of the starting bell at a race, focus your mind and energy with a few moments of deep breathing. Likewise, when you feel you might blow a gasket with your kids, your boss, or the traffic, remind yourself to breathe and the situation will pass.

BREATHING DURING YOGA PRACTICE

In all yoga practice, it is crucial to incorporate yogic breathing. Review the breathing techniques detailed in this chapter. Either sitting or standing on your yoga mat, begin your yoga practice with a few rounds of ujjayi breathing. If you establish the rhythm and flow of the breath at the outset, you will find it easier to maintain during the physical practice.

As a general rule, inhale to move into a pose and exhale to come out of a pose. There are three phases to each pose:

1. Moving into the pose: Inhale.
2. Being in the pose: Count the desired number of breaths.
3. Coming out of the pose: Exhale.

It is important to breathe through each of the three phases. During your time in the pose, take the recommended number of breaths deeply and fully before coming out of the pose and moving to the next one.

Ideally, an even flow of breath is maintained through the entire practice. However, if the pose or sequence is challenging, the tendency is to hold your breath, which is completely counterproductive. Gasping for breath or taking short, shallow breaths indicates that you are struggling in the pose. At any time you can stop, move into a calming pose such as equal standing or child's pose, regain control of your breath, and resume your practice.

You can practice breathing techniques alone for their sole benefits, and you will experience tremendous benefits from combining breathing with the physical practice of yoga. Over time, the depth and ease of the breath will naturally increase, as will your lung capacity. Becoming familiar with your breathing patterns on your yoga mat will give you greater insight and awareness about your breathing while you are running. While the breathing techniques used in running and in yoga are different, the aim of both is to maintain an even and rhythmic breathing pattern and maximize the oxygen intake to fuel your body through the physical demands.

Chapter 4

A Fit Mind

If you are like many people, a typical day may involve arising to the annoying alarm clock, perhaps rustling the kids out of bed, attending to morning hygiene, grabbing something to eat on the run, meeting work demands and the related stresses of achieving and meeting deadlines, rushing home, pulling a meal together, and having a little downtime. Oh yes, and somewhere in this schedule you may have managed to get in a run. During your run you may have mulled over the problems of the day, chatted with running buddies, or listened to music to take your mind elsewhere.

Even your downtime may not really be downtime because it likely includes catching up on e-mails, watching your favorite TV show, or using one of the many electronic devices that keep us connected. You may even keep your cell phone at your bedside so you can be ready to respond instantly. With such a hectic schedule, you may rarely find time to be with yourself, to check in with what is going on in your mind, to take a break from external stimuli, and to be alone and simply be. The thought of being alone with only your thoughts may even be terrifying, or you may simply consider it boring or tell yourself you don't have time.

This chapter explores the idea of not making efforts to accomplish, achieve, or escape from anything. It addresses the concept of just being and experiencing the present moment with awareness and without judgment. This is called mindfulness, and it can be applied to many activities, including physical activity. A mindful approach to any of your activities may be very different from the approach you normally take.

UNITING THE MIND AND BODY

The 1980s defined the fitness craze and led to the birth of a number of exercise varieties, Jazzercise being one of the first. This is also when Jane Fonda's workout videos emerged and led to a variety of aerobics classes, many integrating dance moves performed to music and including quick-paced directions from instructors. The focus of these workouts was exclusively physical, promising toned and sculpted bodies and weight reduction. In addition to issuing instructions, instructors would also shout phrases of encouragement such as, "Keep it moving," "Two more," and "Make it burn." Of course, there were spin-off benefits such as improved self-image and self-empowerment, but the operative aspect was physical exercise.

The 1990s saw a decline in aerobics classes and a greater interest in running and less physically stressful, low-impact forms of exercise. In addition, interest in a more integrated approach to the physical and mental aspects of exercise increased. Thus began the exponential growth cycle of more mind-centered exercises such as yoga, Pilates, and tai chi. People were drawn to exercise programs that focused on the mind and spirit in addition to the physical. During this time the term *mind–body,* which was originally used in the field of medicine (Archer 2004), was applied to fitness. According to the Benson-Henry Institute for Mind Body Medicine in Massachusetts (2013), "Mind-body medicine is based on the inseparable connection between the mind and the body—the complicated interactions that take place among thoughts, the body, and the outside world" (para. 1).

Today, most people acknowledge the positive effect exercise has on mental health, enhancing mood and reducing anxiety and depression (Association for Applied Sport Psychology, n.d.). Because the mind and the body are connected, they affect each other.

Mindfulness and Exercise

Mindfulness can be applied to even the most mundane tasks and can bring about heightened awareness and other positive outcomes. Let's say you have had a stressful day at work and are mulling over matters on your drive home. You literally move into auto pilot and ruminate about the events of the day, perhaps becoming more agitated in the process. In this way you are trapped in the past, lose the present moment, and are unaware of what is happening around you. You may be in the kitchen preparing dinner while caught in the vortex of past deliberations. Once again, you miss out on the present moment and become blind to what could otherwise be a pleasant experience. You don't hear the birds chirping outdoors, you don't take notice of the beautiful flowers on the table, or you fail to notice the vibrancy of the vegetables you are chopping.

Applying mindfulness to even the smallest of tasks can enhance your mood and make you more alert. Most important, it teaches you to stay in the moment rather than letting it fade into the past.

As described by Thich Nhat Hanh in his book *The Miracle of Mindfulness*:

> If while washing dishes, we think only of the cup of tea that awaits us, thus hurrying to get the dishes out of the way as if they were a nuisance, then we are not "washing the dishes to wash the dishes." What's more, we are not alive during the time we are washing the dishes. In fact we are completely incapable of realizing the miracle of life while standing at the sink. If we can't wash the dishes, the chances are we won't be able to drink our tea either. While drinking the cup of tea, we will only be thinking of other things, barely aware of the cup in our hands. Thus we are sucked away into the future—and we are incapable of actually living one minute of life. (1987, 4)

In the fitness world, *mind–body* is used to describe "physical exercise executed with a profoundly inwardly directed focus" (Archer, 2004, para. 9) and is mostly applied to forms of yoga and Pilates. The term *mind–body* refers to a synthesis of the physical and mental aspects of fitness.

Fitness centers often focus on the purely physical aspect of exercise, sometimes offering distractions to purposely take the client's mind from the activity at hand. For example, most gyms have television monitors installed by exercise equipment so clients can be entertained while working out. This separates the mind from the body. Rather than being in touch with your bodily sensations, you move into a robotic state while your mind is transported elsewhere. Some centers lure clients with the promise of changing their body shape so they can fit into skinny jeans or get bikini-ready.

Many people hop from one form of exercise to another hoping to find the one that sticks. Why do some people remain motivated while others lose interest? Why do some people love running from their very first stride, whereas others consider it drudgery? Examining the two types of motivation—intrinsic and extrinsic—may be helpful in understanding these differences.

Extrinsic motivation is driven by external factors: rewards, peer pressure, or a performance goal. People who are extrinsically motivated are more likely to lose interest in the sport once they have met their goal, if the goal has proven to be too difficult to attain, or if they believe their performance does not measure up. Perhaps, in spite of the promise, they don't fit into the skinny jeans after all. People are more likely to lose interest when they are driven solely by external factors, as is typical with purely body-based forms of exercise. An example is the long-time runner who was very keen for his wife to start running so they could share an interest. They developed a plan whereby he paid her for every mile she ran. It worked in the very short term, but after some time she lost interest and decided running was not for her.

Intrinsic motivation can be described as an internal drive, being moved to do something. An intrinsically motivated person undertakes the activity for enjoyment, to grow, or to learn. Pleasure and contentment are gained from the experience of exercising with less emphasis on the outcome. Further, the person feels satisfied with her performance and personal improvement, rather than comparing her performance to others'. Mind–body forms of exercise, which emphasize being in the moment, are more likely to fall into this category. Perhaps this is one reason the tradition of yoga and meditation is considered a practice. Regardless of the number of years engaged in the discipline, there is no measureable goal. The practice itself is the goal.

Examining motivation is familiar among athletes. "Sports psychologists have learned that intrinsic feelings—perceptions of autonomy and competence—are the most powerful motivators, while the promise of a pot of gold actually has the potential to generate *amotivation*. The best way to ensure steady motivation is for athletes to identify effort with something personally satisfying and meaningful. A sense of purpose carries an athlete the farthest and helps him weather the worst storms" (Eliot 2005, 8).

A mind–body focus emphasizes the experience, being present and aware during the activity. With a greater intrinsic focus, you experience the positive feelings related to the exercise and your body and mind are more apt to want to reexperience them. Furthermore, this approach increases the likelihood of continuing with the activity because you are more intrinsically motivated and not focused solely on reaching a goal. When the motivation, or purpose and intention, of the exercise comes from within, you experience internal awareness, also known as mindfulness. As defined by Jon Kabat-Zinn, "Simply put, mindfulness is moment-to-moment awareness. It is cultivated by purposefully paying attention to things we ordinarily never give a moment's thought to. It is a systematic approach to developing new kinds of wisdom in our lives, based on our inner capacities for relaxation, paying attention, awareness, and insight (1990, 2)." In other words, mindfulness means directing attention to the experience in the present moment.

When mindfulness is applied to an activity, it can become a form of mind–body exercise, as illustrated in figure 4.1. Depending on the approach taken, exercise can be categorized as purely physical or as a mind–body experience, and many can be either.

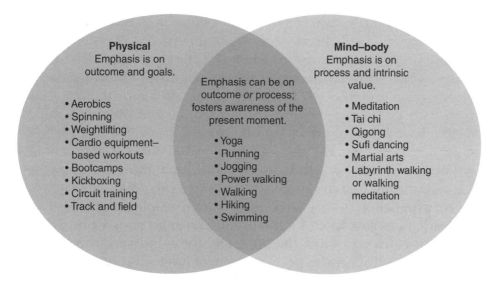

Physical
Emphasis is on outcome and goals.

- Aerobics
- Spinning
- Weightlifting
- Cardio equipment–based workouts
- Bootcamps
- Kickboxing
- Circuit training
- Track and field

Emphasis can be on outcome *or* process; fosters awareness of the present moment.

- Yoga
- Running
- Jogging
- Power walking
- Walking
- Hiking
- Swimming

Mind–body
Emphasis is on process and intrinsic value.

- Meditation
- Tai chi
- Qigong
- Sufi dancing
- Martial arts
- Labyrinth walking or walking meditation

▶ **Figure 4.1** Categories of exercise.

Exercise is physical when the emphasis is solely on an outcome or goal (e.g., to increase speed or strength to gain approval or recognition). The following points describe exercise that is physically based:

- Is extrinsically motivating
- Uses highly charged, fast-paced, loud music to pump up the energy
- Intentionally distracts the mind

Exercise that is mind–body oriented focuses on intrinsic value and an awareness of the process; it uses little or no metric. The following points describe exercise that is mind–body focused:

- Is mindfully executed
- Is intrinsically motivating
- Coordinates movement with the breath
- Encourages people to be with, and enjoy, the experience
- Does not involve judgment, measurement, or comparison to others

Many forms of exercise can be either physically or mind–body focused depending on the person's approach. Exercise done solely for a physical purpose (to lose weight or improve running time) can become a mind–body experience when the emphasis is on the process and it fosters an awareness of the present moment.

You may be surprised to see yoga in the "either" category. Without question, yoga was traditionally a mind–body discipline. The asanas, or physical postures, were merely a means of preparing the body for periods of sitting still in meditation. Adapted to the Western world, yoga has undergone a transformation to fit the needs and tastes of our society, which values outcomes. We are taught to evaluate ourselves by comparing ourselves to others and against standards that have little to do with our direct experience or personal meaning and values. Western yoga has evolved within this cultural context. Thus, yoga can be practiced on a purely physical basis and in some instances looks and feels much like an aerobics class with loud music for distraction or entertainment and the promise of a yoga body. Alternatively, yoga can be experienced solely as a mind–body discipline with the focus on breath and meditation. It can also be experienced as a blend when the breath is used to unite the body and the mind and people strive to remain mindful, in the present moment, and nonjudgmental even during a challenging physical practice.

Running can also be either a purely physical workout or a mind–body experience. Running can be highly social, uniting people sharing a common purpose and including chatter and communal gatherings. For those who run alone, technology has made it easy to take music along; many runners can't get through a run without being plugged into their playlists. Running gadgets abound, too, and many runners are wired with equipment to measure time, distance, heart rate, and pace. They try to run faster and longer, and they monitor their heart rates while they're at it. Then they repeat the next day and compare their performances.

Many runners need the goal of an organized race to give their running a purpose and to maintain their motivation. Races themselves, although providing a sense of satisfaction, can also be a source of stress and dissatisfaction when race goals are not met. Some runners are obsessed with timing their runs, constantly seeking to improve and being disappointed and frustrated when they don't beat their previous times. Running in this manner becomes extrinsically focused and disconnects the mind from the body.

Runners often seek to be entertained rather than feel the physical sensations of the body and the related mental response. Furthermore, because the sport is largely goal oriented, many drop out. It is easy to burn out, lose motivation, or get caught up in the competitive aspect of running so that it becomes another source of stress. As described by road racer turned ultramarathoner Carla Cesaroni: "I stopped running road marathons because it became too much about the time, equipment, etc., and it was destroying my love of running. I came within 2 minutes of qualifying for Boston, but by that time I had learned to hate running." (pers. comm.)

Mindfulness and Running

Running as a mind–body exercise is approached differently than running to achieve a goal. Running with mindfulness—being in the present moment—allows you to directly experience whatever is arising in your field of awareness, without creating an elaborate narrative in your mind about the experience. When running in a mindful way, you do not seek to be distracted from the experience, nor do you try to push the experience away. As described by Laurisa Dill, a runner who practices mindfulness while running:

> *"When I ran my first marathon I was in trouble just after I hit the 21 km mark. I was exhausted, my quads were burning, and my mind was telling me that this wasn't going to happen. Mindfulness was the stance of ever-so-slightly being on the periphery of those internal sensations and thoughts . . . experiencing and watching the mind and the body. Practicing patience, acceptance, and staying present and in the race, I continued to put one foot in front of the other, without being overwhelmed, panicked, or dropping out of the race. Without pushing these sensations out of my mind, I was able to adjust my pace accordingly and went on to finish the race. By being mindful, I didn't overidentify with the experience, thoughts, and sensations, nor did I try to escape the experience." (pers. comm.)*

Running offers tremendous physical and mental benefits, contributing to fitness and overall health and well-being. Most runners are adept at hard measures such as time, distance, and pace and at taking their minds elsewhere while running. Runners are less adept at monitoring the mental responses to running, or at applying mindfulness to their running. Rather than let running be strictly a physical exercise, why not decide to run mindfully, turning it into a mind–body experience, truly a meditation in motion? You could focus on enjoying your time in your moving body without the need to be faster or to train for a race. Rather, you could consider the time you spend running as a date with yourself, with no expectations or judgments.

Make it a point to practice mindfulness during at least one of your weekly runs, and be open to the experience. Following are some suggestions to get you started.

While running, be more in tune with the external environment. When possible, select a route where you can be in nature (e.g., a local park, a field, or a trail), and take note of the scenery—the trees and flowers you are passing. Depending on the time of day, notice the shadows created by the light; sunset and sunrise can be especially magical. Try some trail running to be truly in nature and for a different experience.

Even urban settings offer much beauty to enjoy—the architecture, the storefronts, the lawns and gardens of houses you run by. Take note of the rich colors in both urban and rural settings. Be in tune with sounds, be they birds, traffic, or people. Be in the moment, aware of your internal experience—the feeling of your feet on the pavement, the shirt on your back, and the sweat beads forming on your brow; the sound and feel of your heartbeat; the sound and rhythm of your breath; and the feel of the air as it enters and leaves your body. Now remain focused on your thoughts and where your mind is wandering. Bring it back and decide to be present for the enriched experience that may arise. What is your mood? Are you counting the steps until you are done, or are you able to enjoy each footstep with complete disregard for the miles gone by or yet to be run?

Become passionate about running for the experience, for the time you spend with yourself, and not for the outcome. There are so many beautiful discoveries to be made about your body and mind and the world around you. The beauty is that you don't need to do anything except pay attention. Through evolution, your body knows just what to do, so as you put one foot in front of the other, just experience the moment. Your body will fall into a rhythm, and your mind will fall into a meditative state. There is no need to *do* anything . . . just be.

Even and tempered breathing is vital for runners. You can learn to stay in tune with your breath by observing its tendencies. Try to synchronize it with your stride. If your breathing becomes choppy and erratic, slow down and try to make it even. If it's even and controlled, pick up the speed and observe how the pattern changes.

Many runners keep running logs and monitor their distances, times, and other metrics. If you are a log keeper, consider including some reflections on your internal experience. How easy was it to remain focused during your run? What thoughts kept entering your mind? How did your body feel after the run? How did your mind feel? Did you learn anything about yourself? Did you enjoy the run? Are you looking forward to the next run?

If you are accustomed to running with a group, run solo, at least some of the time. Leave your gadgets behind. Run a familiar route and don't time it. Reinforce to yourself that it doesn't matter how long it took, and try to eliminate expectations. Aim to enjoy the run rather than think about any particular goal. Experience the moment and witness what unfolds.

All elite and world-class athletes spend as much time training their minds as they do their bodies. They incorporate meditation, visualization and psychological training so they are prepared to approach their sports with mind and body. Such practices are crucial for performing at the top of their game. Witness the leading pack of runners in any race, be it a marathon or a sprint. Their bodies are relaxed and in control, moving with grace and efficiency while their facial features reflect their determination and single-mindedness. Athletes performing at their peak do so with mindfulness and every ounce of their energy and mental focus aimed at the task. They are in the zone, completely and wholly immersed in the activity. If you are an amateur or casual runner, you may simply go out for a leisurely jog rather than striving for a high-level performance, yet you, too, can explore the benefits that mindfulness brings.

Bringing mindfulness to the activity may very well improve the experience, and the results may be surprising. From an overall health and wellness perspective, there is undeniable value to be gained from integrating the mind and body and, in so doing, uniting physical and mental fitness.

MEDITATION

Practicing mindfulness helps cultivate a broader awareness of your experience. When you are mindful, you are more likely to have a holistic approach in which you experience a unification of mind and body. When you are mindful, you can recognize your experience, your pain, your suffering, your happiness, and your pleasures as part of an interdependent system that includes your mind, body, and environment. One of the simplest ways to cultivate this holistic perspective is through meditation.

The recent explosion of interest in yoga has ignited a greater interest in meditation. Yet, meditation itself has been in practice since ancient times, often as a form of religious ritual such as prayer, chanting, singing, and reflection. Practices such as meditation and yoga are known as *contemplative practices,* meaning that they are practiced to emphasize awareness and to set one's intentions to a broader purpose.

Meditation is the practice of concentrating your focus on one thing such as a sound, a candle flame, or your breath so you can be in the present moment, rather than being in the past or projecting into the future. Traditionally, the physical practice of yoga was done to prepare the body for meditation. When you have excess energy or are fatigued or stiff, sitting in one position for a period of time without becoming fidgety can be difficult. A physical yoga practice energizes the body while settling the mind, making it a perfect preparatory activity for meditation.

Benefits of Meditation for Runners

Our society operates at a frenetic pace—meeting deadlines, achieving results, getting things done only to move onto the next item on a to-do list. Perhaps this is the root of the rise in interest in meditation. Once you experience the inner calm and settling of the mind that meditation offers, if even for a moment, you may seek to revisit that state time and again. Much scientific research has been done on meditation, and although the results may vary, most experts agree on the following benefits:

Stress Reduction   Meditation is understood to be one of the best methods for reducing stress. Excessive stress can create an imbalance in your nervous system, keeping you in the fight-or-flight mode; meditation reduces stress by activating your body's natural relaxation response. Simply by quieting and settling your mind, you can put aside the myriad of worries that plague you. By spending time alone in contemplation and in the present moment, you become more relaxed, resulting in reduced stress levels. Through the relatively simple act of observing your inner state, your breath, and your thoughts, you may find that many of your nagging worries are actually quite trivial. In this way you learn to let go of the little things and appreciate what is important in life.

Incorporating meditation into your running may bring exciting results. It may change your relationship with running and provide a completely new outlook on it. It can also heighten the mental benefits of running while eliminating the stress-inducing aspects of it.

Better Health   Stress is harmful to health and is responsible for a range of problems affecting individuals and society at large. It contributes to many physical ailments such as heart disease, high blood pressure, chronic fatigue, sleep disorders, ulcers, and headaches. It also contributes to psychological distress, insomnia, mood swings, and anxiety attacks.

Meditation is a powerful tool for reducing disease and restoring physical and mental health. Because of the relationship between mind and body, the peace of mind that meditation instills can resolve many stress-related ailments.

As a runner, you already gain tremendous physical benefits from running; introducing meditation into your running will augment these benefits by taking care of your mind. The mind and body, acting as one, create a greater overall sense of well-being.

Concentration   Meditation greatly improves concentration, which is imperative for meeting life's daily demands. With greater concentration, you can work more efficiently because you are less distracted, and you can better channel your energy to the task at hand. Professional athletes also use meditation. Studies have shown that improved concentration improves athletic performance (Jha, et al. 2007). The ability to solve problems and make decisions is also enhanced when the mind has greater clarity.

Meditation eliminates or reduces the chatter and clutter of the mind. With a single point of focus, all unnecessary thoughts are put aside. Applying meditation to your running will increase your focus and concentration, which can lead to greater satisfaction; it may also, surprisingly, improve your results. Many runners have experienced a time when the power of concentration and focus has helped them cross a finish line!

A Stronger Mind   While strengthening your body with physical exercise, you also need to strengthen your mind to achieve mind–body harmony. Meditation can be viewed as a psychological exercise that will reward you with improved concentration and a stronger mind. Through meditation you can control the fluctuations of the mind. When the mind is under more control, it is better able to guide you through life. Research at UCLA (2009) has shown that those who meditate actually have certain regions of the brain that are larger than those regions in people who do not meditate; this enhances their ability to concentrate deeply and react to life's situations with greater emotional stability.

It is truly a win–win–win situation when running develops your physical strength and cardiorespiratory capacity, yoga further balances and strengthens you, and meditation strengthens your brain. Strength of mind and mind control are also extremely helpful during a race!

Contentment   Everyone wants to be happy. However, many seek that happiness from external sources or create conditions for happiness (e.g., "I will be happy when . . ."). Through the inner peace of mind that meditation brings, you may discover a self-generated sense of contentment, without conditions. In fact, research shows that meditation can actually rewire the brain to be happier. Meditating with a focus on appreciation or gratitude creates powerfully positive emotional responses (Ricard 2006).

You may feel disappointed when you don't meet your race goals, your running pace does not meet your expectations, or you fail to qualify for a desired race. Shifting the focus to meditative running opens the door to finding greater contentment with your efforts, regardless of the outcome. You may even feel euphoric after a run, even if it was a slow one!

Living in the Present   The thinking mind lives in the past or the future. When you are in those states, you miss out on the opportunity to be in the present. In fact, being present, or practicing mindfulness, allows you to see and experience what is right in front of you. Through meditation you learn to be in the present moment, initially during your time in meditation but eventually in other activities of daily life. Being in the present moment reduces the pondering or obsessing over problems, and you are more apt to appreciate some of the surrounding beauty and blessings in your own life. There is wisdom in the adage that reminds you to stop and smell the roses.

If you are like many runners, you may often look at your watch and calculate how much time, or how many miles, remain. If you are having a bad run, you can't wait for it to be over. Meditative running brings you into the moment to experience the good; you may realize that what you thought was bad is actually good. Being present while running gives you the opportunity to experience the benefits of running with every stride and with every breath: the energy pumping through your body, the feeling of being alive, the feeling of freedom, your heart pounding to greater strength.

Intuition   You have no doubt experienced gut feelings or moments of inspiration when ideas or solutions to nagging problems jump into your mind. This is intuition, that inner voice that guides you, that sixth sense that is so difficult to define. Whether you recognize it or not, you use intuition in daily life. However, your intuitive sense is easily drowned out by the hectic pace of daily living and the many demands on your time and energy. Through the power of meditation, the distractions are reduced and you can become more aware of your inner self and better able to discern the internal messages. The more you acknowledge your intuition, the stronger it becomes, and you learn to listen. By quieting the mind and being in the present moment, as you are in meditation, your intuition improves. Listening to that inner voice may even save you from incurring injuries: If those hamstrings are speaking to you, don't ignore the message! Remember that intuition only exists in the present moment.

Patience   We live in a fast-paced world and are accustomed to moving through it at breakneck speed. As a result of fast food, fast cash, and instant messaging, the mind is trained to expect instant results. This creates impatience and even rage when things are not delivered quickly—for example, while waiting in line or stopped in traffic. The ability to remain calm and centered from within helps you cope with situations that would otherwise create stress. The mere act of sitting, doing nothing, and being in a state of being rather than doing, as in meditation, gives you greater patience. Improved patience, with yourself and with others, makes you more tolerant and more tolerable.

When you are impatient, you may be eager to get what is before you out of the way so you can move on to the next thing; in this way, you are projecting into the future. This easily transfers to running; from the first few moments of your run, you may be anticipating the end of it by counting the miles or the time. Adopting a meditative approach to running instead helps you enjoy your time running. Even when you face a challenge, such as a big hill, you can remain focused and connected with your breath and patiently make your way up the hill. You can then enjoy the ease of running on a flat surface.

The Meaning of Life Meditation is a tool that helps in exploring the profound question about the meaning of life. We are trained to look for meaning in life by societal values such as our income, our success, our possessions—mostly external markers. Through meditation you gain a deeper understanding of who you are, on the inside, and gain a broader perspective as you begin to recognize that all events and actions are part of a larger interdependent world. Feelings of emptiness can be replaced with a sense of abundance; feelings of longing can be replaced with a sense of gratitude. By changing your perspective of yourself, you may experience changes in your relationships and find yourself moving toward greater contentment. Meditation and mindfulness can help you stay connected to your core values and what you want your life to stand for.

Exploring the meaning of life can also help you understand the role running plays in your life. Running provides a vehicle through which you can learn a tremendous amount about yourself. It is easy to be content and satisfied when you meet your running goals, but what you learn about yourself when you face disappointments is more profound. For example, how do you deal with slower race times than you hoped for, or an injury that derails your running? What happens when an injury prevents you from running the race with the friends you have trained with, or you feel a sense of failure when you lose your motivation to keep running? Although running can add richness to your life, is it what defines you as a person?

The Meditation Process

You can approach a meditation practice in many ways, including taking courses, listening to CDs, or investigating the myriad of reading material on the topic. Whichever method you select, be aware that results do not come instantly. It is called meditation practice because you need to keep doing it to reap the benefits. Meditation is not something you do for a period of time, understand, and move on from. It is a lifelong practice that cannot be measured by daily results. It is not something you need to do perfectly. The aim is to simply commit to doing it daily, do the best you can, and let the results seep into your life, which may happen in subtle, yet powerful ways.

The best approach to beginning a meditation practice is to simply start with no expectations. Simply give yourself to the experience. Following are some basics to get you started.

Prepare Your Space

As detailed earlier, you can introduce meditation into your running for the added benefit of turning it into a deeper mind–body experience. You can integrate it into your yoga practice for a more mindful and richer experience. You can also practice it while doing the simplest of tasks, like sorting laundry, cooking, or washing the dishes. However, at times you may simply want to meditate—that is, be still and experience the moment. Perhaps you are experiencing an especially stressful time in your life, feel overwhelmed, are on an emotional roller-coaster, or simply feel the need to check in with yourself. Setting aside some time and an appropriate space in your home can help you rejuvenate and calm your mind. Additionally, sitting and meditating will sharpen your ability to integrate mindfulness into both your running and your yoga practice.

Space Create a space in your home that is quiet, tidy, clean, and free of distractions such as people and sounds. Keep anything that will remind you of something on your to-do list out of site (e.g., laundry). The space can be small, but it should be pleasant and inviting. Add a pleasant smell if you like by burning incense or a candle.

Do Not Disturb Physically and mentally establish a "do not disturb" time and space. Even in the middle of a busy household, create peaceful practice conditions and be sure you won't be disturbed. Leave all electronic devices, including your cell phone, in another room.

Time Set aside a time daily. The body and the mind respond well to routine, so if possible, set aside the same time every day. Start small by setting aside 10 minutes as your time to meditate. You can lengthen the duration as you gain comfort and ease.

Prepare Your Body

The typical image of someone in meditation is sitting on the floor, legs entwined in a full lotus position. For many of us, this is a far-fetched dream and is certainly not a prerequisite for meditation. The most important thing is to be comfortable, which varies by individual.

If your body is stiff and sore, you will have difficulty sitting still. Even if you force yourself to do so, you will likely not look forward to doing it again. Thus, it is advisable to take a few minutes to prepare your body by doing some simple stretching. The time spent doing some preparatory yoga poses will also help your meditation by bringing your attention to your body and starting your mind moving inward.

Sitting on the floor is easy, connects you more directly to the earth, and encourages you to sit upright. Sitting upright in a natural and comfortable position with the chest open makes it easier to breathe deeply. Sit on a mat, blanket, or rug in a simple cross-legged position and elevate the hips by sitting on a pillow (figure 4.2). This allows the hips to tilt forward and makes it easier to maintain a tall spine.

If sitting on the floor is too challenging at the outset, sitting on a chair is fine; however, try to sit forward with your feet on the floor and your spine upright. If you can, refrain from relying on the chair back. Regardless of your sitting preference, hold your spine upright and keep your shoulders relaxed with your head resting comfortably on your shoulders.

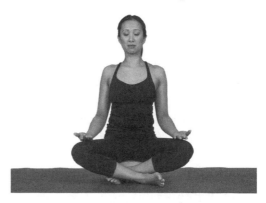

▶ **Figure 4.2** Sitting on the floor is the most typical body position for meditation.

How to Meditate

While meditating, your eyes can be closed or open, whichever makes you feel more at ease. With eyes open it is helpful to have an object to focus on: a candle flame, a crystal, or a flower. The purpose of the item is to be a focal point to strengthen your attention when it wanes; it's less important what it is. With eyes closed, create an internal point of focus in the darkness. It can be the image of a flickering candle flame or a colored dot.

The breath can also be a focal point for meditation. Start by examining your breath using mindful observation. Listen to the sound of the breath, feel it enter each nostril, and follow its path through the nasal passage and into the lungs. Observe how the lungs respond to the breath by expanding the chest; exhale and feel the chest retract. Observe the rhythmic ebb and flow of the breath.

Maintain focus and attention on your point of meditation. Thoughts and distractions will enter your mind or your mind will start to wander to some external place. Do not let your thoughts take root—simply put them aside for the moment. Without judgment, bring your mind back to your focal point. Keep in mind that such distractions are completely normal; when they occur, remain calm and, without judgment, simply return to your focal point, either the visual object or your breath. Regardless of how frequently your mind wanders, just bring it back and continue.

Even after just a few minutes, your body will start to object and your mind will focus on the little aches and pains emerging, or that itch that just needs scratching. Try to remain still and again bring your mind back to your focal point. Eventually, those physical distractions will transform or shift. With practice, the quiet time between thoughts and distractions will grow.

Although on the surface, meditation sounds simple, it is not. Do not set unrealistic expectations because they will lead to a feeling of self-defeat. Furthermore, don't expect magnanimous changes or spiritual enlightenment to take place. The benefits will reveal themselves in subtle ways over time.

The key to meditation is to persevere. Stay on the path while acknowledging and accepting the difficult and easy aspects of the practice that arise. At the end of a mediation practice, you may want to extend appreciation or gratitude to yourself for the effort and intention you set to stay present.

REFERENCES

Archer, S. 2004. What is mind-body exercise? *IDEA Fitness Journal,* www.ideafit.com/fitness-library/what-is-mind-body-exercise.

Association for Applied Sport Psychology. n.d. Psychological benefits of exercise. www.appliedsportpsych.org/Resource-Center/health-and-fitness/articles/psych-benefits-of-exercise.

Benson Henry Institute for Mind Body Medicine. 2013. What is mind body medicine? www.massgeneral.org/bhi/basics/whatisMBM.aspx.

Eliot. J.F. 2005. Motivation: The need to achieve. In *The Sport Psych Handbook,* ed. S. Murphy, 3-18. Champaign, IL: Human Kinetics.

Jha, A.P., J. Krompinger, and M.J. Baime. 2007. Mindfulness training modifies subsystems of attention. *Cognitive, Affective, & Behavioral Neuroscience* 7, no. 2 (June): 109-119.

Kabat-Zinn, J. 1990. *Full Catastrophe Living.* New York: Bantam Dell.

Nhat Hanh, T. 1987. The Miracle of Mindfulness. Boston: Beacon Press.

Ricard, M. 2006. Happiness: A Guide to Developing Life's Most Important Skill. New York: Little, Brown.

University of California at Los Angeles. 2009, May 12. Meditation may increase gray matter. News release.

Chapter 5

Running Injuries

You are training for a big race, you are on track with your program, you are having some great runs and are feeling yourself getting fitter by the day, and suddenly you feel a twinge or pain while running. The pain may subside, but it may also be an early sign of an underlying problem. Unlike acute injuries related to some sports, running injuries give the body ample warning signals.

Nothing is more frustrating for a runner than facing an injury. Nonetheless, the reality is that a majority of runners will face an injury at some point in their running careers. The high risk of injury is due to the repetitive nature of running, overusing some muscles and underusing others, compounded by the weight-bearing impact of the sport.

OVERUSE INJURIES

When you run, specific muscles in your legs, hips, and feet are used in continuous repetition and thus can become overused. As a result of being in a constant state of contraction, the overused muscles shorten. Without an opportunity to restore length, these muscles will continue to shorten and eventually restrict and limit the range of motion of related joints, create misalignment in the body, and thereby make you prone to injury.

Running injuries typically occur below the waist and can involve related joints, muscles, tendons, ligaments, and sometimes bones. Most commonly they involve the legs, hips, knees, ankles, and feet. The injuries can be acute, as in stepping in a pothole and straining an ankle, but more common are overuse injuries that develop over time and are caused by an accumulation of physical stress on the body. Although overuse injuries may appear to present themselves instantly, it is more likely that warning signs were present and either ignored or misread. Every runner's hope when experiencing a troublesome signal is to be able to run through it.

Several factors may contribute to overuse injuries, some to do with individual body structure and biomechanical predisposition, and others to do with training method or equipment. Following are key factors that contribute to running injuries:

- Muscle imbalances
- Overly tight or overly lax muscles and joints
- Innate misalignment patterns (such as leg length discrepancy)
- Inappropriate running shoes
- Increasing the mileage, speed, or quality of runs too quickly
- Running repeatedly on uneven surfaces

Although there is no silver bullet to guarantee that running injuries will not occur, there are steps you can take to minimize their risk.

YOGA FOR INJURY PREVENTION

Runners love to run, and to have longevity in the sport, they would be wise to develop a smart plan to mitigate the risk of injury. Taking care of the controllable factors is a good place to start—that is, finding and following a running program suited to your personal running history. Starting with a plan is especially important when you are new to running, as is having the advice and guidance of a supportive running coach or experienced running friend. If you don't have a coach or a friend to advise you, a myriad of training programs and methods are available through books and the Internet.

Next, buy a good pair of running shoes from a knowledgeable salesperson at a runners' shop. Unlike when purchasing general use shoes, which are suitable if they simply feel comfortable, many factors should be taken into account when purchasing running shoes, such as pronation, supination, arch type, and style of running. A knowledgeable salesperson will be able to evaluate your needs and recommend an appropriate shoe. Not only does this ensure that your money is well spent, but it is also key to injury prevention and comfort.

So now you have a plan, have purchased a suitable pair of running shoes, and are all set to start your program. But have you considered incorporating a way to reduce the risk of injury into this program? Knowing that many risk factors are associated with the physical stress of running and muscle imbalances, you need to counter these risks.

Runners are generally eager to get on the road and deal with injuries only when they occur. A safer and smarter strategy, and one that is more likely to help you meet your overall fitness goals, is to integrate injury prevention into your program at the outset.

Yoga is a perfect complement to running, and integrating a yoga practice into your weekly fitness plan is an excellent way to safeguard against injuries. As detailed in chapter 2, in addition to eliminating those nagging aches and pains that like to settle into the body, yoga can prevent and heal injuries.

Yoga immediately reveals and addresses the muscle imbalances that often lead to injury. By its very nature, yoga helps restore the body to balance and symmetry. Runners who take part in yoga are often surprised to discover the differences in strength and flexibility between their right and left sides. Likewise, many make the unexpected discovery that they have a weak upper body and core and learn that this can contribute to injury. But often most astonishing is the discovery that their legs may be strong for running but not overall, because they have not developed strength in all muscle groups.

Take a simple lunge, for example. It is not uncommon for runners new to yoga to be very unstable and shaky in this pose, doing all they can to stay upright and not fall over, rather than being grounded through the feet, stable in the legs, and strong through the torso with straight arms extended overhead and breathing deeply and calmly. The position of the legs in a basic high lunge may seem very similar to a running stride, but a running stride involves movement; the lunge is static, meaning that you can't escape the work. During a lunge all the muscles in the legs, as well as the ankles and feet, are either contracting or stretching.

When executed with correct alignment and attention to detail, the high lunge holds many benefits for runners:

Bent Front Leg

- Strengthens the hamstrings
- Strengthens the ankle
- Strengthens the gluteus medius
- Strengthens muscles of the front shin
- Strengthens the inner quadriceps
- Stretches the outer quadriceps

Straight Back Leg

- Stretches the sole of the foot
- Stretches the ankle joint

- Stretches the Achilles tendon
- Stretches the calf
- Stretches the hip flexors

Torso

- Lengthens the spine
- Strengthens the abdominals
- Strengthens the muscles of the upper back
- Stretches the shoulder muscles
- Improves the range of motion of the shoulder joint

Overall

- Improves balance
- Improves focus and concentration

Lunges can be very challenging for runners at the beginning. However, the balance of strength and flexibility they develop reduces the risk of a number of injuries. Additionally, as runners improve in their performance of the lunge, their running strides lengthen, they move with greater ease, and their athletic performance improves. Finally, remaining in the pose for a period of time requires the focus of mind and will, as does successfully crossing the finish line at a race. And these are the benefits from merely one pose! Compound this effect with the number of yoga poses done in a full yoga practice, and the results are truly astounding.

A yoga practice, especially one designed to meet the specific needs of runners, reduces the risk of injury. A yoga practice that focuses on proper alignment with a balanced blend of stretching and strengthening is ideal. Furthermore, practiced mindfully with appropriate attention to detail and accompanied by deep diaphragmatic breathing, yoga offers the tremendous mind–body benefits described in chapter 4.

Whether you have been running for years or planning your very first run, integrating yoga will benefit you. It is never too late to start a yoga practice, and there is no such thing as being too stiff for yoga. Many runners turn to yoga when they have had an injury and use it as a way to recover. When the symptoms subside, they consider themselves cured and return to their previous routines, but often the injury returns and then they return to yoga.

Rather than using yoga on an irregular, as-needed basis, integrate it into your program on an ongoing basis by making time for it in your weekly workout. Think of it as putting money in the bank for that rainy day, and perhaps you will help to ensure that the rainy day will never come. Approached in this manner, yoga will keep your body strong and balanced for running and for the physical demands of everyday life. Moreover, like interest in your bank account, the benefits of yoga compound over time. Even after only a few weeks of regular practice, many students feel stronger and more limber and are able to bring increased body awareness to their running. Additionally, it is not uncommon for runners who have started a yoga practice to run faster, set new personal bests, and then wonder whether yoga had something to do with it.

Nicola's Story

I had run three marathons, including Iron Man and Boston, and was training for my fourth. It was a fund-raiser taking place in Ireland, where I am from, so many friends and family were planning to cheer me on. I was running 60 miles (97 km) per week and feeling good, except for some nagging hip and lower-back discomfort that I thought, or hoped, would go away with physio treatments. However, the pain got worse, becoming so intense that running was out of the question. I was in a state of depression seeing this goal vanish.

A friend suggested yoga, and luckily I found *Yoga for Runners*. I was completely new to yoga and surprised at how stiff I was. I thought yoga was OK, and at least it gave me something physical to focus on while not running. I did five yoga classes per week for two weeks with no running. I was feeling better and did a few short runs. About five weeks prior to the marathon, I started some longer runs, but throughout kept doing yoga a few times a week. The pain was virtually gone, but I was fearful it would return if I pushed it. Compared to my previous training, I felt undertrained, but decided I would try to run the race anyway and not care about time. At the beginning of the race, I felt very relaxed. To my astonishment, I had a very strong finish and ran a personal best time of 3:08.

My pain was in the lower back, hip, and sciatica. Reflecting on my experience, I know the injury was a result of years of training hard and doing no stretching to speak of. Yoga completely loosened my hamstrings, which then loosened my hips and lower back. My upper body felt stronger as well. My stride completely came back, and my whole body felt much less stressed. I felt great overall, body and mind. Yoga saved me, and I will always make time for it in my training.

RUNNING INJURIES AND YOGA

As you now know, the primary cause of running injuries is overuse—the repeated pressure on the body, stride after stride, day after day. The good news is that you can prevent many running injuries by being alert to the signals your body sends you and then taking action before an injury develops. Following are the most common running injuries:

- Knee pain
- Shin splints
- Plantar fasciitis
- Achilles tendinitis
- Flat feet
- Iliotibial band syndrome (ITBS)
- Hip pain or strain
- Hip weakness
- Sciatica
- Hamstring strain or pull
- Groin strain or pull
- Lower-back pain
- Upper-back or shoulder tightness or pain
- Side stitches

Furthermore, the cause of running injuries can be categorized as follows:

- Muscle tightness
- Tendinitis
- Muscle weakness
- Muscle imbalance

As explained earlier, yoga is an effective way to keep the body in balance and in tune for healthy and pain-free running. A balanced yoga practice, mindfully executed, will go a long way in helping you avoid or minimize these common causes of running injuries and the injuries themselves.

There are yoga miracles, such as a nagging issue that resolves after only one yoga class. For example, a long-time runner may be experiencing pain in the knee from a tight iliotibial band and after one yoga class be suddenly pain free. Cases such as this are clearly the exceptions, but it is not uncommon for students to feel an ease in lower-back tightness after only one or two yoga classes. Most commonly, students express simply feeling better, stretched out, and calmer.

Although feeling better instantly is a good way to keep a runner on a yoga mat, it must once again be stressed that the greatest benefits are gained over the long term. As the tight muscles stretch out and the weak ones strengthen, the body achieves greater balance and symmetry. In addition, greater body awareness and improved posture transfers to better body carriage while running and performing daily tasks. It is over time and as a result of a regular practice that the deeper and greater rewards are experienced.

A balanced and consistent yoga practice is the best way to keep your body tuned up. If you are dealing with a specific injury, some yoga poses should be included in your recovery plan. See table 5.1 for a list of common running injuries, poses that address them, and how yoga helps.

Yoga can help the full spectrum of running injuries. No muscle in the body works in isolation. Rather, all movement requires the coordinated effort of various muscles and joints so that the body moves as an integrated whole. Because it stretches muscles, improves balance, and strengthens the body, yoga is the perfect companion to running. Given the cardiorespiratory benefits of running, combining it with yoga is the best road toward a complete and integrated fitness plan.

Table 5.1   Common Running Injuries and How Yoga Helps

Injury	Anatomical condition	How yoga helps	Poses
FEET, KNEES, AND LOWER LEGS			
Knee pain	*Runner's knee* is a general term for a variety of disorders caused by various factors; often it is an overuse injury created by a biomechanical irregularity that occurs when the kneecap is out of alignment as it tracks over the thigh bone. Leading causes are muscular imbalance or misalignment in the feet, ankles, and hips or muscular imbalance of the inner and outer quads.	• Stretches overly tight quads • Strengthens inner quads • Strengthens hip stabilizers • Decompresses knee joints • Strengthens core	• Quadriceps and IT band rollouts • Hero pose • Wall squat • Lunges • All standing poses, with focus on contracting quads when legs are straight • Gluteus medius–strengthening exercises • Equal standing, where all weight bearing joints are in alignment

(continued)

Table 5.1 (continued)

Injury	Anatomical condition	How yoga helps	Poses
FEET, KNEES, AND LOWER LEGS (CONTINUED)			
Shin splints	Overuse injury in which the tendon and adjoining tissue of the tibia are inflamed, with tenderness, pain, and sometimes swelling experienced along the mid- to lower shin.	• Stretches calves. • Stretches and strengthens shins • Strengthens arches of feet	• Downward dog • Hero pose • Squat • Lunges
Plantar fasciitis	Inflammation of the plantar fascia, a broad band of connective tissue along the bottom of the foot; pain is most commonly felt at the heel; will start as a bruised sensation and if not treated will become a sharp, stabbing pain.	• Stretches calves • Stretches soles of feet • Strengthens arches of feet	• Hero toes • Downward dog • Plantar massage
Achilles tendinitis	Inflammation of the large tendon at the back of the ankle; symptoms range from swelling and tenderness to sharp and severe pain at the lower ankle; if left untreated, can rupture.	• Stretches calves • Strengthens calves • Strengthens ankle joints • Balances strength in leg muscles	• Hero toes • Foot extension and flexion work • Balance poses • Downward dog • Lunges • Squat
Flat feet	Cause of foot pain that can affect running stride and contribute to knee pain, shin splints, Achilles tendinitis, and plantar fasciitis.	• Strengthens muscles of feet • Reduces lower-leg weight impact by strengthening the core and hips	• Toe spreading • Hero pose • Hero toes • Standing poses, with emphasis on lifting arches and inner ankles
Iliotibial band syndrome (ITBS)	A thick band of tissue (fascia) extending along the outer hip and thigh and inserting below the knee acting as a stabilizer of the hips, legs, and knees, which becomes inflamed and irritated from overuse.	• Stretches hamstrings • Stretches quads • Increases mobility of hip joint • Stretches tight glutes • Strengthens abductors	• Gluteus medius–strengthening exercises • Supine hamstrings stretches • Revolved triangle • Internal rotator stretch • Half frog • Kneeling quad stretch • Iliotibial band and quad rollout • Supine twist
HIPS			
Hip pain or strain	Can come from any of the pelvic joints (hip joints, sacroiliac joints, pubic symphysis) and may relate to the tendons, bursa, and any of the muscles that attach to the pelvis.	• Increases range of motion of hip joint • Stretches external rotators • Stretches internal rotators • Strengthens hips • Strengthens core	• All hip-opening poses • Standing poses • Gluteus medius–strengthening exercises • Iliotibial band rollout

Injury	Anatomical condition	How yoga helps	Poses
Hip weakness	Common among runners because the gluteus muscle group is not used as much as other muscle groups while running; affects lower-extremity biomechanics and can lead to any number of injuries of the lower limbs.	• Strengthens gluteus medius • Strengthens gluteus maximus. • Strengthens hip abductors • Stretches overly tight glutes	• Gluteus medius–strengthening exercises • Tabletop with extended leg • Downward dog–leg extended variation • Internal rotator stretch • Lunges • Standing poses • Balance poses
Sciatica	Caused by pressure on the sciatic nerve or herniated lumbar vertebra from tight lower-back muscles and tight external hip rotators, especially the piriformis.	• Stretches piriformis • Stretches back muscles • Decompresses spine • Stretches hamstrings	• Downward dog • Pigeon • Double pigeon • Knee to ankle balance • Chair hip stretch
Hamstring strain	A very common running injury resulting in pain in the back of the thigh, often leading to a strain or tear of the hamstring tendon and creating pain at the sitting bone or the back of the knee; caused by tight and weak hamstrings.	• Stretches hamstrings • Strengthens hamstrings • Stretches quadriceps • Balances hips	• Standing poses • Supine hamstrings stretch • Straight-leg lunge • Revolved triangle • Quad stretch • (*Note:* Proper hamstring stretching is crucial because of the high risk of injury as a result of overstretching. During poses that stretch the hamstrings, the focus should always be on stretching the belly of the muscles to avoid straining the hamstring tendons.)
Groin strain or pull	Pain in the upper inner thigh, usually caused by tightness in the adductor muscle (although it can be a sudden injury due to running on a slippery surface or speed work).	• Stretches inner thighs • Increases mobility of ankle joints • Stretches the hip flexors	• All wide-leg standing and seated forward bends • Bound angle • Lunges • Standing poses, with inner thighs contracting
LOWER AND UPPER BACK			
Lower-back pain	Caused by any biomechanical imbalance that affects the lower back; pain is mostly felt in the lumbar region and typically is the result of muscular strain or spasm; also caused by tight back muscles and tight hamstrings.	• Stretches tight back muscles • Strengthens back muscles • Strengthens core • Stretches hip flexors • Stretches hamstrings • Balances musculoskeletal system • Improves postural alignment	• Downward dog • Half downward dog • Child's pose • Legs up the wall • Overall yoga practice, including stretching, strengthening, and twists

(continued)

Table 5.1 (continued)

Injury	Anatomical condition	How yoga helps	Poses
LOWER AND UPPER BACK (CONTINUED)			
Upper-back or shoulder tightness or pain	Mostly caused by lifestyle factors leading to tension and tightness held in the upper body and characterized as shoulders lifted to the ears with a rounded upper back.	• Strengthens upper-torso musculature • Relaxes upper traps • Increases body awareness • Strengthens core	• Upper-body strengthening • Plank • Chaturanga • Dolphin (downward dog variation) • Dolphin plank • Shoulder stretches
OTHER			
Side stitches	A sharp, intense pain under the lower edge of the rib cage as the result of a muscle spasm of the diaphragm brought on by shallow chest breathing.	• Deepens diaphragmatic breathing • Elongates torso and improves overall breathing • Strengthens core to improve running posture	• All yoga poses • Diaphragmatic breathing

Chapter 6

Feet, Ankles, and Knees: Stabilize Your Foundation

All standing structures need a foundation, and the stronger the foundation is, the more stable the structure will be. This is especially important under adverse conditions that would otherwise topple the structure. Whether the structure is a house, a high rise, or a bridge, the visible component is what impresses us, but the most vital part of the construction is what we don't see.

Evolutionary theory explains why and how humans evolved from moving on four legs (quadrupeds) to two (bipeds). However, there is no doubt that quadrupeds have far greater stability than bipeds. As you move through your daily tasks, the many advantages to having a solid and stable foundation are clear. Runners need to be solidly grounded when their feet touch the pavement. To achieve this, the feet, ankles, and knees need to not only be strong, but also mobile and flexible to provide the propulsion to move forward.

This chapter explores the most fundamental aspect of your foundation: the feet, ankles, and knees. Your feet are what connect you to the earth, grounding you and giving you the necessary gift of stability. As we will explore in subsequent chapters, other physical factors contribute to overall stability, but it starts with the feet. Yet, many of us abuse our feet. Certainly, we take them for granted—at least until a problem develops.

STRUCTURE OF THE FOOT AND ANKLE

The average runner strikes the ground 1,000 times per mile with a force of two to three times his body weight. The feet and ankles take the brunt of this impact, because they are the first point of contact with the ground. The ability to maintain strength and balance while hitting the ground affects the entire body. Additionally, because feet and ankles are structured to act as shock absorbers, it is particularly crucial for runners that they be in shape.

To support the body while standing, walking, or running, the foot and ankle structure needs to be stable and flexible. Stability is necessary for supporting body weight and maintaining balance, and flexibility is necessary for propelling the body forward. Healthy feet and ankles are crucial to athletic performance and overall well-being. Although you may be able to continue running with tight hamstrings or a sore hip, most foot problems will stop you in your tracks.

The foot and ankle contain the following:

- 26 bones (one-quarter of the bones in the human body are in the feet)
- 33 joints
- More than 100 muscles, tendons (fibrous tissues that connect muscles to bones), and ligaments (fibrous tissues that connect bones to other bones)
- A network of blood vessels, nerves, skin, and soft tissue

The foot and ankle joint is amazingly strong, given the weight-bearing work it assumes. Yet, as a result of overuse, neglect, and abuse, this structure can experience nasty injuries at some point in a runner's career. Furthermore, a problem in the foot or ankle can create problems elsewhere in the body—namely, the knees, hips, or spine.

The Foot

We don't often think about exercising our feet. Rather, we allow the joints and ligaments to become stiff and immobile and the muscles to atrophy. Consider the state of muscles after being confined in a cast to heal a broken bone: They become visibly shrunken and noticeably weaker after just a few weeks. This is basically the same effect on the musculature of the feet, except it is compounded by years of being crammed into shoes, losing muscle tone, and losing the ability to move freely. As with other parts of the body, the muscles and joints in the feet need to be exercised to be healthy, functional, and happy.

From a very young age, we are accustomed to wearing shoes. We may cram our feet into fashionable shoes with little regard for the long-term effect. Constrictive shoes restrict blood circulation in the feet and compress the bones. Compounding that effect is the fact that we wear shoes for hours on end day after day, taking little or no time to exercise our feet. Modern-day foot problems such as bunions, hammertoes, and weak, or fallen, arches are the result of this type of neglect.

Most footwear pushes weight forward to the balls of the feet, which causes some muscles and tendons to weaken from underuse. High-heeled shoes worsen the situation, placing the calves and related tendons in a state of contraction and shortening them over time. Simply walking barefoot makes use of the muscles of the feet and lower legs and helps to keep the muscles and tendons toned. In addition, it allows the toes to spread and the feet to be unrestricted. Recall the wondrous feeling of walking barefoot on a warm, sandy beach!

Additionally, we tend to keep our feet covered and hidden most of the time, so we are less likely to be aware of the more subtle, yet key, changes in their structure and appearance. Because the feet are the body's foundation, the arches are crucial in providing stability and agility. They provide a natural air sole and act as shock absorbers while walking and running. The arches are maintained by the bone structure and supported by the ligaments, muscles, and tendons in the feet. Weak, or fallen, arches can be painful, hinder stability, make walking difficult, and lead to problems in the knees and lower back.

Following are the three arches in the foot (figure 6.1):

Medial longitudinal—The highest arch and the one we are most familiar with. It extends along the inner foot from heel to big toe.

Lateral longitudinal—A lower and flatter arch than the medial-longitudinal arch. It extends along the outer edge of the foot from the outer heel to baby toe.

Transverse—This arch is a little more mysterious, and one we may not be aware of. It extends across the width of the foot, at the base of the toes.

Assessing the health of your arches is a simple process. When coming out of a swimming pool or bath, place your foot on a dry surface and examine the shape created. A healthy arch will show an imprint along the outer foot, while the inner foot section is clear. A fallen arch will show an even imprint along the entire surface. A high arch will show only a thin strip along the outer foot.

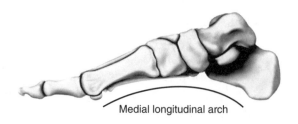

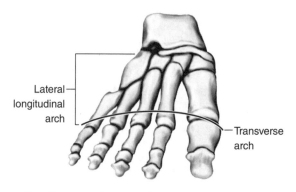

▶ **Figure 6.1** The three arches of the foot.

Although some people are born with flat feet, in most cases the condition develops in adulthood. This is typically the result of wearing tight footwear that compresses the joints or high heels, which place the weight at the toe bases and cause a strain on the arches.

The Ankle

The ankle is a hinge joint, and its unique structure requires a balance of strength for stability and range of motion to permit walking and running. The ankle joint (figure 6.2) is composed of the following:

Tibia and fibula—The lower leg bones.

Talus—The foot bone.

Ligaments—Structural support.

The range of motion of the ankle joint is created by the muscles of the lower leg, whose tendons cross the ankle and attach at the foot. Movement is created through the contraction of the leg muscles, permitting us to walk or run. Along with the foot, the ankle joint also functions as a shock absorber.

The hinge action of the ankle joint creates its primary movements of flexion, extension, and rotation. An efficient running stride requires a sufficient degree of mobility in the ankle joint so you can push off the toes to move forward. Additionally, you need sufficient range to accom-

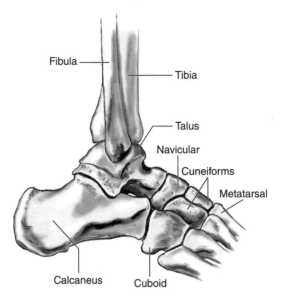

Fibula

Tibia

Talus

Navicular

Cuneiforms

Metatarsal

Calcaneus

Cuboid

▶ **Figure 6.2** The ankle joint.

modate uneven surfaces. In addition to limiting the range of motion in your stride, overly stiff ankle joints are more easily susceptible to strain. For example, a common twisted ankle injury is caused when the rotation of the ankle joint is beyond the range of motion of the joint, as may occur as a result of stepping in a pothole or rolling off a curb. An overly tight ankle joint is more easily susceptible to sprain, torn ligaments, or even stress fracture.

RUNNING, YOGA, AND THE FOOT AND ANKLE

As described earlier, the feet take a beating by being in shoes all day, and running only exacerbates the related compression and tightening. Aesthetically, running can create calluses, blisters, and black toenails. Running can cause painful toes, ball joints, heels, and ankles. Functionally, tight feet and ankle joints can affect overall biomechanics and running form. As with all joints, the ankles need to maintain a reasonable range of motion to propel the body forward during a running stride. Similarly, the joints in the feet need strength and flexibility to provide balance while walking and running and to provide thrust for the gait. The feet and ankles are the first in line to be affected by the repeated weight-bearing action of running, and you would be wise not to ignore this crucial part of your anatomy.

In yoga, the feet and ankles are of the utmost importance. Yoga is always done in bare feet, primarily to allow you to feel the ground and also to give the feet freedom to move with no unnecessary restrictions. Some people new to yoga wear socks and are shy about going barefoot and exposing their feet. Runners with black or missing toenails, calluses, or blisters are often horrified at the thought of being barefoot.

Virtually every yoga pose requires the foot to perform a specific action. A typical yoga practice involves moving the ankle joints through their intended range of motion of extension, flexion, and rotation. You have the opportunity to strengthen the feet as you learn how to lift the arches throughout the standing poses, stretch the bottoms of the feet, and relearn how to mobilize the toes by curling, extending, and spreading them. Mostly this is done merely as a result of properly executing the yoga pose. In fact, the emphasis of the pose may actually be elsewhere (e.g., in the hips), yet the feet and ankles work to accommodate the setup and alignment and stabilize you while you hold the pose.

In addition to having a well-rounded yoga practice, you can do exercises that deal specifically with the feet. Proper alignment, which you seek in your yoga practice, involves bearing weight evenly at three points of each foot: the big toe base, the baby toe base, and the center of the heel. Many foot problems cause unevenness in the grounding of the feet, resulting in the weight rolling inward or outward or too far forward or back on the foot. That is, rather than being evenly distributed through the sole of the foot, the weight is unevenly distributed. This type of misalignment in the feet has repercussions throughout the entire body. As the most fundamental component of your stability, misalignment in the feet affects your knees, hips, and spine.

YOGA POSES FOR THE FOOT AND ANKLE

As discussed in previous chapters, yoga is a practice that involves all parts of the body and the mind. In this chapter and the four that follow, a specific body focus or benefit is assigned to each pose. However, it is important to keep in mind that the holistic nature of yoga requires mindfulness and for all parts of the body to perform their functions.

Following are yoga poses that benefit your base—the feet and ankles.

Equal Standing

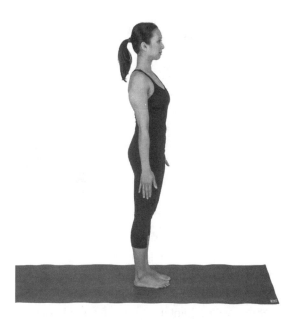

Description

1. Stand with feet together and the inner edges of the big toes touching. Lift and spread the toes, pressing the big toes toward each other and fanning the other toes outward.

2. Align the weight-bearing joints, with the head over the shoulders, shoulders over the hips, hips over the knees, and knees over the ankles.

3. Press down evenly through the base of the big toe, base of the baby toe, and center of the heel. Feel an even distribution of weight on the right and left foot.

4. Without rolling the weight to the outer feet, lift the inner ankles to activate the inner (medial longitudinal) arches.

5. Contract the quadriceps, especially the inner quadriceps, and feel the kneecaps lift.

6. Broaden the collarbones and press the shoulder blades down and into the back.

7. Lift the breastbone (sternum) and draw the front ribs in.

8. With solid grounding of the feet and support of the legs, lengthen the upper body from the base of the spine to the crown of the head.

Benefits

- Is a fundamental pose
- Aligns the body toward balance and symmetry
- Is an excellent off-the-mat pose that can be practiced anytime you are standing
- Creates awareness of postural habits
- Strengthens the thighs, knees, ankles, and arches of the feet

Plantar Massage

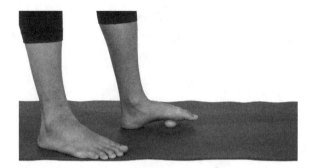

Description

1. Start in equal standing, with feet hip-distance apart.
2. Place a small, hard ball under the cuboid bone on the outer edge of the foot. Press the foot down, using full body weight if possible. Hold for 5 breaths.
3. Place the ball at the big toe joint and press down. Hold; then repeat, moving the ball to each joint. Hold for a few breaths at each joint.
4. Place the ball at the base of the big toe joint and slowly roll the foot on the ball lengthwise to the heel, pressing your body weight into the ball. Slowly move the ball to the next toe joint and repeat.

Benefits

- Massages the soles of the feet
- Breaks down scar tissue and lesions related to plantar fasciitis
- Relieves tired feet
- Improves circulation to the feet
- Stimulates pressure points relating to the entire body

Simple Balance

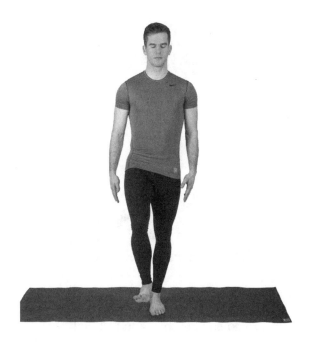

Description

1. Start in equal standing, with feet hip-distance apart.
2. Close the eyes and lift the right foot a few inches off the floor. Keep the eyes closed. (*Note:* If unable to maintain balance with eyes closed, start with eyes open and close the eyes as balance improves.)
3. Repeat on the other side.

Benefits

- Strengthens the ankles
- Improves balance

Hero Pose

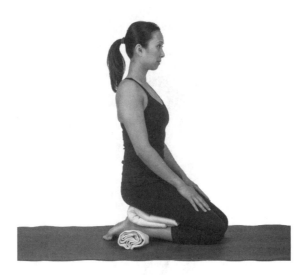

Description

1. Use a folded blanket to pad the shins and feet. If the ankles or tops of the feet hurt, place a rolled blanket at the instep for support. If unable to sit on the heels without knee pain, place a folded blanket or bolster between the hips and the feet.

2. Kneel on the floor with the knees and big toes touching. The shins and tops of the feet are flat on the floor. Spread the toes so that all the toes touch the floor.

3. Sit back so the sitting bones rest on the heels.

4. Sit upright with the shoulders over the hips and the head over the shoulders, lengthening the spine from the sacrum to the crown of the head.

5. Do not overdo this pose. Hold only as long as is comfortable, increasing the length of time slowly. This pose should be done daily for best results.

6. At first, the heels will splay outward. Over time, start to bring the heels toward each other so that the inner and outer ankles are equal in length.

Benefits

- Strengthens the arches of the feet
- Increases flexibility of the ankle joints
- Stretches the shins
- Decompresses the knee joints
- Stretches the quadriceps
- Encourages good posture, because it is very difficult to slouch in this position

Hero Toes

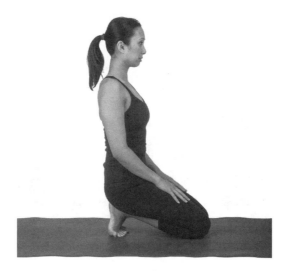

Description

1. Start in hero pose. Lean forward and take the hands to the floor in front of the knees
2. Keep the knees on the floor and curl the toes under, including the baby toes if possible
3. With toes curled under and heels lifted to upright, sit back onto the heels
4. If there is intense pain, lean forward to ease the weight in the feet. Otherwise, sit tall with the shoulders over the hips

Benefits

- Stretches the soles of the feet, including the plantar fascia
- Mobilizes the toe joints
- Improves circulation to the feet

Toe Spreading

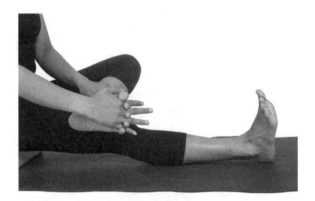

Description

1. Sit on the floor or on a block with the legs straight.
2. Bend the left leg and place the ankle on the right thigh. Insert the fingers of the right hand between the toes, taking the webbing of the hand to the webbing of the toes.
3. Move the toes forward and backward, squeeze the fingers with the toes, rotate the ankle in one direction and then in the other, and finally alternate between pointing the toes and flexing the foot.
4. Remove the fingers and spread the toes.
5. Repeat with the other foot.

Benefits

- Increases flexibility and mobility in the toes
- Increases the range of motion of the ankle joints
- Offsets the formation of and pain related to bunions

STRUCTURE OF THE KNEE

The knee joint is quite simple in its function as a hinge, yet the structure is complex and somewhat delicate. The knees are very susceptible to injury because they serve a crucial role in weight bearing, which is compounded during the actions of walking, running, climbing, and squatting. Thus, it is no surprise that knees are more likely to be injured than any other joint in the body. Among runners, knee problems and risk of injury occur most frequently.

The knee (figure 6.3) is made up of four bones:

Femur—The thigh bone. It is the largest, longest, and one of the strongest bones in the body. At the bottom, it is part of the knee joint, and at the top, it meets the hip bone to create the hip joint.

Tibia—The second-longest bone and the larger of the two bones that make up the lower leg. It connects the ankle to the knee, and its primary functions are for movement and weight bearing.

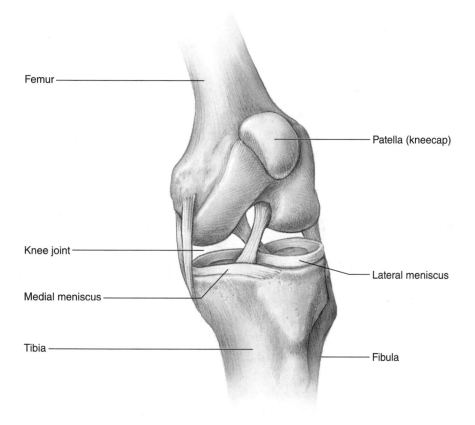

▶ **Figure 6.3** The knee joint.

Fibula—The smaller of the two lower leg bones that runs parallel to the tibia. Its main function is for stability, particularly of the ankle joint.

Patella—The kneecap. It sits on the femur, and its main function is extension, sliding whenever the leg bends. It also protects the knee joint.

The bones of the knee joint are covered by cartilage, which acts as a buffer to prevent the bones from rubbing together. In addition, there are two C-shaped pads between the tibia and the femur, known as meniscus, which further cushion the joint, absorb shock, and ease weight bearing in the joint. Two main tendons attach to the knee, the iliotibial band and the quadriceps. A number of ligaments support and stabilize the knee, much like the trusses of a bridge. The ligaments are key to the structure of the knee joint, because they provide support, literally holding it together during various movements. In a healthy knee joint, the femur and tibia are properly aligned, the patella tracks smoothly through movement, and the weight is evenly distributed at the inner and outer pads of the meniscus.

As a hinge, the knee joint has a rather simple movement pattern: bending (flexing) and straightening (extending). There is only a slight rotational range of movement in the knee joint. The muscles that directly support and facilitate knee movement are the quadriceps at the front of the knee and the hamstrings at the back. The quadriceps straightens the leg (extension), and the hamstrings bend the leg (flexion).

To be healthy, knees need the supporting muscles to be balanced in strength and flexibility and the cartilage and ligaments to be strong and smooth. Problems can occur when any of the components of the knee joint are under stress, aggravated, or damaged. Additionally, the knee joint is often the innocent victim that suffers as a result of misalignment at the hips, feet, and ankles or weakness of the supporting quadriceps.

RUNNING, YOGA, AND THE KNEE

Knee injuries are one of the most common among runners. Sports that require quick changes in directional movement, such as soccer and baseball, have a high risk of acute ligament injury. For runners, knee problems typically arise over time; the nagging discomfort that comes and goes, if not dealt with, can lead to more serious problems. Knee injuries can arise from overtraining and are typically related to misalignment, muscle weakness, or muscle tightness.

Proper alignment includes a vertical lineup of the hip, knee, and ankle joint. As a relatively simple hinging joint, the knee has problems when the tracking of the bone structure becomes misaligned. Misalignment in the feet, ankles, or hips will have an impact on the knee. Pronating (rolling the foot in) or supinating (turning the foot out too much) while running or walking decreases the stability of the knee joint. When the feet make an incorrect movement every time they hit the ground, the constant pounding and repetition manifests in the knee. Likewise, an imbalance in the hips affects the knees through the related movement of the femur bone.

Another cause of knee pain for runners relates to the iliotibial band (IT band), a fibrous band of fascia that extends from the top of the hip bone and attaches on the tibia below the knee. The IT band's role is to stabilize the knee while walking or running. In runners, the IT band becomes tight from overuse and overly tight leg muscles and is felt as pain in the outer knee.

Additionally, runners tend to have tight outer quads and weak inner quads. This imbalance creates a torquing action in the knee, which pulls the kneecap and twists it to the side so the patella no longer tracks as it should; over time this creates pain and wears down the cartilage around the knee. This is generally referred to as runner's knee. In addition, simple wear and tear from weight bearing can affect the cartilage of the knee bones and lead to inflammation and arthritis.

It is easy to see that muscle or skeletal imbalances in any number of areas can have a detrimental effect on our precious knees.

Yoga can be both a curse and a blessing for the knees. With proper instruction and awareness, yoga is the perfect aide to restore the balance and symmetry required for proper knee alignment. A yoga routine can include poses that specifically focus on aspects of the knee, but more important, it helps restore the entire body to balance and symmetry, which returns the knee to a state of balance.

However, yoga can also create knee problems or aggravate existing issues if poses are performed improperly. The knees are at the greatest risk in hip-opening poses and in standing poses. In standing poses, knee alignment must be correct and the required muscles must be contracted to support the knee structure so that the weight-bearing element strengthens the muscles without disturbing the knee joint.

In seated or supine hip-opening poses, the desired movement *must* come from the hip joint. Problems occur when the hip joint is tight and limited in its movement. Pushing beyond where your hip mobility allows torques the knee past the limited rotational capacity of the knee joint and stresses it. For example, when sitting in a simple cross-legged position on the floor, your knees may be quite high off the floor (well above the waist). The distance of the knees from the floor relates to the range of motion of the femur bone at the hip joint. If you try to lower the knees by pushing down on them, you will exert harmful pressure at the knee joint, specifically the meniscus. The knee joint is much weaker and more fragile than the hip joint, so it will be the first to take the strain. Unless these actions are done to the extreme, there is no immediate pain, which only encourages you to keep doing it. Then, after some time, you wonder why your knees are hurting.

Another common alignment issue in yoga is hyperextending the knee joint (i.e., pushing the knee back when standing). Many people believe they are simply straightening the leg, but in fact they are pushing the knee joint too far back and out of proper tracking alignment. This is particularly common in those with lax joints. This repeated action causes pain at the back of the knee. The best way to avoid hyperextension of the knee joint is to contract the quadriceps.

You need to be particularly mindful of the alignment of the knees in standing postures and even more mindful that hip opening remains centered at the hip joints. During all standing actions, the back of the knees should remain soft and the quadriceps should be contracted. Furthermore, whenever the legs are straight, the center of the knee joint should be aligned with the center of the hip joint and center of the ankle joint.

YOGA POSES FOR THE KNEE

Many of the yoga poses in subsequent chapters will help create healthy knees. Balancing the hips; strengthening and stretching the muscles in the legs and the feet; and improving core strength all have a positive effect on the health of the knees. The poses and exercises in this section are additional remedial work for those suffering from knee issues.

Equal Standing

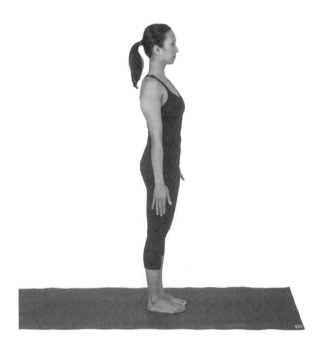

Description

1. Perform the action as described in Yoga Poses for the Foot and Ankle.
2. Keep the hip, knee, and ankle joints in alignment.
3. Contract the quadriceps, especially the inner quads. Ensure that the back of the knees are soft.

Benefits

- Strengthens the inner quadriceps
- Balances the strength of the inner and outer quadriceps
- Encourages proper alignment of the lower body

Wall Squat

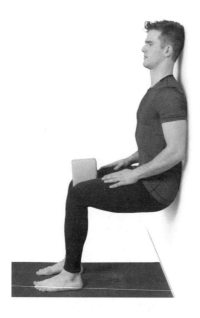

Description

1. Standing in front of a wall, bend the legs and rest the upper body at the wall; then walk the feet forward until the legs are at 90 degrees.
2. Align the feet so they are parallel and hip-distance apart, and keep the knees over the ankles. It may be helpful to place a yoga block between the knees and press the inner knees into the block. Do not let the knees splay; keep them directly over the ankles.
3. Press evenly into the feet, as in equal standing.
4. Contract the hamstrings to support the knees.
5. Press the lower back into the wall and keep the head upright.
6. Correct alignment is crucial. It is helpful to do this exercise in front of a mirror to be certain of feet and leg alignment.

Benefits

- Strengthens the inner quads
- Stretches the outer quads
- Strengthens the hamstrings
- Promotes proper alignment

Half Frog

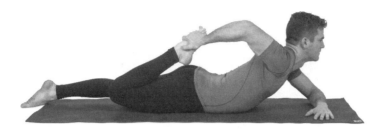

Description

1. Lie prone with the legs extended. Press the front hip bones to the floor.
2. Bend the right leg and take the right hand to the top of the foot. Press the heel toward the right buttock, keeping the hip bone grounded.
3. Place the left arm in front of the body, press the forearm to the floor, and lift the chest.
4. Repeat on the other side.
5. Ensure a stretch is felt in the quadriceps with no pain or extreme tugging action at the knee joint.

Benefits

- Stretches the quadriceps and psoas major
- Strengthens the back muscles

Quadriceps and Iliotibial Band Rollouts

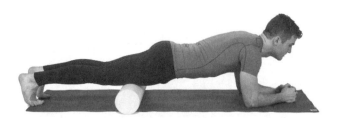

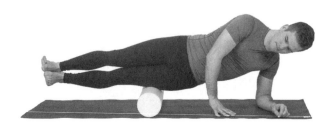

Description

1. Lie prone on a foam roller, placing the roller under the quadriceps.
2. Press the forearms into the floor and roll forward and back, sliding along the roller from the top to the bottom of the thighs. Do not roll over the knees or hip joints.
3. Repeat several times.
4. Roll to one side and continue rolling along the side of the upper thigh for a deep massage effect on the iliotibial band.
5. For both rollouts:
   - Start with the feet resting on the floor, but eventually bring the feet off the floor with both legs straight.
   - As you roll out the length of the front and sides of the thighs, you will likely encounter one or two spots that are particularly painful. Rather than avoid such a spot, remain here, release your body weight into the roller, and allow the tight spot to soften.

Benefits

- Releases tightness in the quadriceps and iliotibial band
- Soothingly self-massages tight muscles
- Increases the flexibility of muscles that attach to the iliotibial band
- Breaks down the tiny lesions that form between the muscles and the fascia

Chapter 7

A Healthy Spine: Reduce Pain, Strain, and Pressure

A key factor in your overall health is a healthy spine. A healthy spine has strong bones and muscles, has flexibility to move freely, and is free of pain. In fact, the spine is the most important component of your well-being, because it houses the central nervous system, which controls and coordinates your movements. As anyone who has suffered from back problems knows firsthand, back pain can deeply affect our quality of life. Keeping your spine healthy is an absolute must if you want to run pain free and remain active.

When the spine is injured and its function is impaired, the consequences can range from being mildly annoying to being chronically painful or physically disabling. It is estimated that 80 percent of the North American population will experience lower-back pain at least once in their lifetimes. To meet the physical demands of running, you must have a strong and healthy spine.

STRUCTURE OF THE SPINE

The spine is the central axis of the skeletal system, allowing you to stand upright while protecting the spinal cord. It is made up of a set of bones called vertebrae. The strong bone structures of the vertebrae protect the more delicate makeup of the spinal cord in the same way that the skull protects the brain. The spinal cord is a column of nerves that connects the brain to the rest of the body and serves as master control over both the physical and mental aspects of your body and mind. The complex and highly coordinated communication system among the brain, the central nervous system, and the peripheral nervous system controls the various body functions such as movement, sensations, memory, and speech.

The Spinal Column

The vertebrae of the spinal column are separated by intervertebral discs (figure 7.1), which are like jelly donuts, a gelatinous core surrounded by a fibrous ring. These intervertebral discs provide cushioning between the bone structures, and their malleability gives the spinal column its mobility and flexibility. The intervertebral discs, along with strong ligaments that run the length of the spine, help unite the bodies of the vertebrae into one strong, structural unit. Healthy discs are plump so they can act as shock absorbers while providing cushioning between the vertebrae to facilitate movement.

The spine is literally the backbone of your structure and extends from the skull to the pelvis (figure 7.2). The 33 individual vertebrae stack on top of each other and are grouped into five segments, as shown in table 7.1.

Cervical Spine (C1–C7) The cervical spine is made up of seven vertebrae and creates an inward C curve at the back of the neck. This region of the spine has the greatest amount of flexibility and is therefore easy to strain if not protected by strong neck muscles and proper alignment. Its main purpose is to support the head, which weighs about 10 to 12 pounds (4.5 to 5.4 kg). In neutral spinal alignment, the head is positioned on its axis and perfectly balanced in its place. Some lifestyle

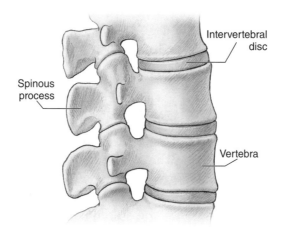

Intervertebral disc

Spinous process

Vertebra

▶ **Figure 7.1**　Vertebrae and intervertebral discs.

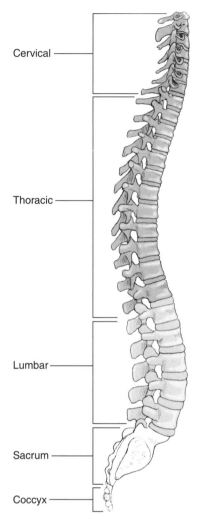

Cervical

Thoracic

Lumbar

Sacrum

Coccyx

▶ **Figure 7.2**   The spinal column.

Table 7.1   Segments of the Spine

Segment	Number of vertebrae	Body area	Conventional abbreviation
Cervical spine	7	Neck	C1–C7
Thoracic spine	12	Chest	T1–T12
Lumbar spine	5	Lower back	L1–L5
Sacrum	5 (fused)	Pelvis	S1–S5
Coccyx	3-5	Tailbone	None

factors (such as working at a computer, using handheld devices, and driving) cause the head to tilt forward on its axis for many hours at a time, causing imbalance and strain on the spinal column.

Thoracic Spine (T1–T12)   The thoracic spine provides attachment points for the rib cage that serve to protect the vital organs. At T11 and T12, the ribs do not attach to the sternum or costal ridge and are therefore called floating ribs. This segment of the spine creates an outward C shape and is more limited in its range of motion because of the rib–vertebra connections and the shape of the vertebrae. Lifestyle factors—namely, sitting at computers for hours on end—can greatly alter the natural C-shaped curve of the thoracic spine and create a stooped effect: an overly rounded thoracic spine with the chest caved in.

Lumbar Spine (L1–L5)   The lumbar spine, or lower back, has the important job of bearing the body's weight. As a result, the lumbar vertebrae are larger than the others. The natural curve of the lumbar spine creates an inward C shape. Next to the cervical spine, this region is the most mobile. The lower back is often overly tight and compressed, making it easily strained by lifting heavy items, twisting while carrying weight, or even simply carrying heavy objects. The lower back is the most common area of discomfort and the most at risk for disc herniation. For runners, it is especially important to have a healthy lower back because weight bearing, and the related biomechanical stress, is greatly compounded during the action of running.

Sacrum (S1–S5)   The sacrum is located at the base of the spine and is lodged between the two large pelvic bones connecting the spine to the pelvis. Five bones are fused into a triangular shape to form the sacrum, which attaches to the pelvic bones on either side to create the sacroiliac (SI) joints. These joints can be (and often are) too lax, overly tight, or misaligned, any of which can lead to pain. The sacrum is a key anatomical landmark when describing yoga poses because its movement sets the base for the rest of the vertebrae.

Coccyx   Immediately below the sacrum are three to five additional bones, fused together to form the coccyx, or tailbone. It is an evolutionary remnant of a tail and, although it doesn't have a particular function, it is a very useful reference point in yoga to help direct the movement of the spine.

Back Muscles

In addition to the bone structure and supporting ligaments, a large and complex group of muscles supports the spine, adding to its ability to support the body's weight in stillness while allowing the trunk to move in many directions. The main movements of the spine are flexion (bending forward), extension (bending backward), lateral flexion (bending sideways), and rotation. A healthy spine moves well in each of these directions. Following are the specific muscles that aid in these movements:

Extensor muscles—Attach to the back of the spine and support the ability to stand and lift objects.

Flexor muscles—Attach to the front of the spine and facilitate forward bending, arching the back, and lifting. The abdominal muscles are included in this group and are located in front of the spine.

Oblique muscles—Attach to the sides of the spine and wrap around the rib cage. They support rotation of the spine, allow lateral flexion, and stabilize the trunk.

SPINAL MISALIGNMENT

Although a number of factors may contribute to back problems, good posture is the best place to start to remedy them. Posture is the carriage of the body while standing, sitting, and lying down. You started out with good posture as a child, but as lifestyle factors set in, many of which kept the spine in a sedentary position for hours, misalignments started to occur. Your posture, whether good or bad, is with you every moment of your life. Good posture makes you look and feel healthier while adding to your youthfulness and confidence, and it is the first step to being pain free. For runners, improving posture translates into better running form and a more efficient running stride.

When the body is aligned in proper posture, there is the least amount of strain on the spinal column, supporting back muscles, and ligaments during standing, sitting, walking, running, and other weight-bearing activities. Proper postural alignment helps maintain the natural S-shaped curve of the spine. This curvature makes the spine architecturally strong and resilient, distributing mechanical stress while seated or standing, and during movement. When the natural curves are in place, the spine is strong and gives you the balance and stability you need to stand, walk, and run.

Proper posture also prevents fatigue because muscles are used more efficiently, conserving energy. The bones, muscles, and ligaments of a properly aligned spine move smoothly and are pain free during daily activities and while running. Imbalances in the spine cause further imbalances in other parts of the body as they attempt to compensate.

Following are factors that contribute to poor posture:

- Unawareness
- Excess weight
- Weak abdominal muscles
- Weak upper-body muscles
- Tight muscles
- Wearing high-heeled shoes
- A poor work environment
- Poor sitting and standing habits

It is not uncommon to have some degree of spinal misalignment, which manifests as natural curves that are exaggerated or out of place. Following are the primary types of spinal curve abnormalities (figure 7.3):

Lordosis—Commonly known as swayback, an excessive inward curve at the lumbar spine. This is caused by any number of bio-mechanical imbalances in the hip region or weak abdominals. The natural curve of the lumbar spine can also become flattened. This can be caused by overly tight hamstrings and back muscles as well as degenerative factors such as arthritis.

Kyphosis—An abnormally rounded upper back, causing the head to be pitched forward. Abnormal kyphosis can be caused by poor posture, weak back muscles and ligaments, or a structural condition.

Scoliosis—An abnormal curving of the spine to the left or right side. This condition can be caused by repeated patterns in the body that have caused extreme muscle tightness, resulting in a misalignment of the vertebrae. Congenital scoliosis is a condition from birth. Either can cause great discomfort.

The effect of spinal curvature abnormalities can be relatively minor, causing mild discomfort from time to time. Left untreated over time, however, these patterns can settle into the body until back pain becomes chronic.

RUNNING, YOGA, AND THE SPINE

Running is a weight-bearing sport and creates repetitive stress for periods of time. For some people running creates back pain, especially in the lower back, and there is no question that running will exacerbate an underlying back problem. If left untreated, back pain can become

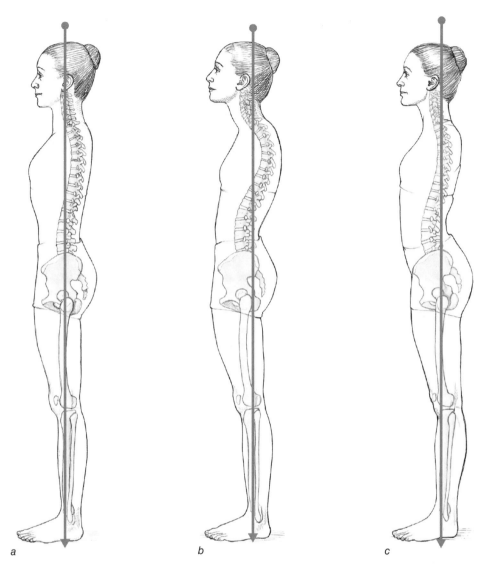

▶ **Figure 7.3** Spinal curve abnormalities: *(a)* neutral spine, *(b)* kyphosis, and *(c)* lordosis.

worse or lead to additional problems in other areas of the body. Proper form while running distributes body weight evenly, rather than loading the lower back with more weight.

It is easy to blame running for lower-back pain, and it does contribute to the problem. However, sitting all day may be the bigger culprit. When seated, especially for an extended period of time, the lower back is sedentary, compressed, and weak. Running simply exacerbates these factors, further compressing and tightening the back.

For healthy running, you need to take care of the spine. Of course, one of the best ways to do this is to integrate a yoga practice into your weekly fitness routine. Yoga will undo the effects of sitting and running by lengthening, strengthening, and realigning the spine.

Although the practice of yoga dates back thousands of years, with the recent growth of yoga, researchers have become more interested in assessing related health benefits. Key among these is yoga's effect on chronic lower-back pain. Results of an extensive study on yoga for back pain, published in the *Archives of Internal Medicine*, showed that 12 weeks of weekly yoga classes improved back function and reduced pain for those with chronic lower-back pain (Sherman et al. 2011). This does not come as a surprise to those who have experienced the benefits of yoga.

Yoga's traditional role was first and foremost a health management system, and paramount to good health was the health of the spine. Virtually every yoga pose involves the spine. A typical yoga practice requires the spine to move in all directions—namely, extending, flexing, and twisting. Therefore, yoga has the potential to benefit the spine in all areas that pose a risk. Yoga poses tone and strengthen the muscles of the torso, increase the flexibility of the spine, and improve spinal alignment. It is not uncommon for those who undertake a regular yoga practice to actually become taller.

A common adage that reinforces the importance of a healthy spine to overall well-being is that you are only as young as the flexibility of your spine. Let's take a look at the specific way yoga works to create a healthy spine.

Musculature The various back muscles are weak and tight in many of us. Yoga stretches these muscles and at the same time strengthens them. In addition, a major contributor to back pain is weak abdominals, and yoga provides ample opportunities to strengthen the core.

Bone Structure As a result of overly tight back muscles, compounded by the weight bearing of sitting, standing, and walking, the spinal vertebrae can become compressed, creating a constant pressure on the spinal discs. Through yoga, the spine is lengthened, relieving the effects of compression. In addition, many styles of yoga, including *Yoga for Runners*, can increase bone strength through weight bearing. The constant contracting and stretching of related muscles increases blood supply to the bones, providing the vital nutrients they require to be healthy.

Posture As mentioned earlier in this chapter, bad posture is a major cause of spinal misalignment. Even after only a few yoga classes, you will become more aware of your posture during your daily activities. This heightened awareness will have an immediate effect on how you carry your body. Furthermore, yoga strengthens postural muscles while stretching those that are overly tight and helps balance the muscles on both sides of the spine. Over time, as the muscles adapt, better posture becomes the norm.

Central Nervous System   While the body movements required for various yoga postures help to tone and strengthen the muscles that support the spine, they also enhance the flow of cerebrospinal fluid within the central nervous system. This effect is enhanced by the deep yogic breathing that energizes the vital fluids in the body, including the cerebrospinal fluid. It is believed that yoga's mind–body benefits may be the result of this increase in the flow of cerebrospinal fluid.

YOGA POSES FOR THE SPINE

All yoga poses have an impact on the spine. In fact, understanding the desired effect on the spine is key to understanding the fundamental nature of the pose. The poses in this section include some basic and essential poses for the spine that bring the benefits of yoga to athletic bodies. Generally, definition of a neutral spine is when the natural curves are in place, creating the desired S shape. Unless otherwise stated, this is the desired shape of the spine while in yoga poses.

Equal Standing, Arms Overhead

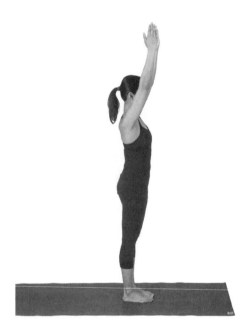

Description

1. Start in equal standing (chapter 6).
2. Roll the upper-arm bones wide, open the palms facing forward, and reach through the fingertips.
3. Slowly take the arms overhead until they are shoulder-distance apart.
4. Keep the arms straight with no bend in the elbows, palms facing each other.
5. Pull the upper-arm bones down so they are secure in the shoulder sockets.
6. Extend through the arms to the fingertips, initiating the stretch from the base of the spine. Keep the feet and legs grounded.
7. Press the shoulder blades down the back and keep the shoulder shelf relaxed (i.e., do not hunch the shoulders).

Benefits

- Stretches the superficial layer of back muscles
- Lengthens the spine
- Stretches the shoulders
- Strengthens the upper back

Standing Side Bend

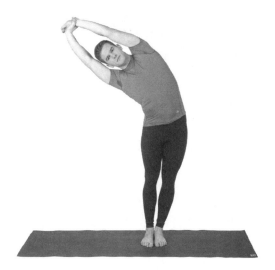

Description

1. Start in equal standing with arms overhead and feet hip-distance apart.
2. Reach for the left wrist with the right hand and bend to the right. As the right arm pulls you to the right, press the left shoulder down.
3. Keep the hips in alignment, facing forward.
4. Keep the feet firmly planted.
5. Hold and breathe deeply into the left side of the body, feeling the rib cage expand with the breath. Try to deepen the side stretch with every breath.
6. Repeat on the other side.

Benefits

- Stretches the obliques
- Stretches the sides of the torso and spine

Half Downward Dog

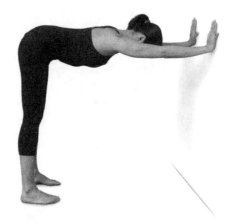

Description

1. Start in equal standing (chapter 6), but with feet hip-distance apart and facing a wall.
2. Place the palms on the wall at hip height, fingers spread and pointed upward.
3. Walk away from the wall, hinge from the hips, and lower the upper body until it is parallel to the floor. Keep the hips over the knees and the knees over the ankles.
4. Straighten the arms and keep the ears in line with the upper arms.
5. Engage the abdominals to support the lower back.
6. Firmly press the hands into the wall and extend the hips away from the wall to lengthen the spine and sides of the torso.
7. Keep the legs straight, quadriceps contracted, and feet firmly grounded.

Benefits

- Stretches the spinal muscles
- Rejuvenates the spinal discs
- Stretches the shoulders and chest
- Stretches the hamstrings and calves
- Strengthens the arms and legs

Cat–Dog Stretch

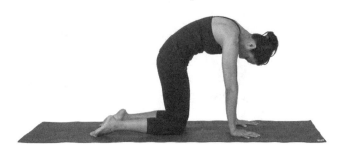

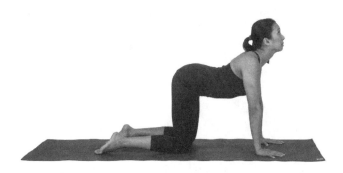

Description

1. Start on hands and knees. Place the hands under the shoulders with fingers spread and hips over the knees. Rest the tops of the feet on the floor. The spine is in a neutral position.

2. Exhale and draw the belly in, lifting the belly button toward the lower back and rounding the back toward the ceiling (cat). Pull the tailbone down. Relax the shoulders and let the head hang.

3. Inhale, release the lower back, lift the sitting bones to the sky, slide the breastbone forward, and gaze to the ceiling.

4. Alternate these actions, coordinating the movement with the breath. To come out of the pose, return the spine to neutral.

Benefits

- Mobilizes the vertebrae
- Gently massages the spine and internal organs

Child's Pose

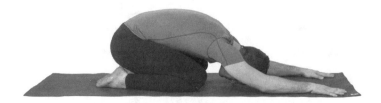

Description

1. Start on hands and knees with feet together and knees hip-distance or more apart.
2. Press the shins and the tops of the feet into the floor and slowly press the hips back, coming to rest with the sitting bones on the heels.
3. Lengthen the upper body, fold forward, and rest the head on the floor or a folded blanket. Arms can be straight and extended forward for a deeper back stretch or bent and wrapped around the thighs for a more relaxing pose.
4. The back should be rounded. Relax the lower back and upper body and breathe deeply, expanding the lower back with the breath.

Benefits

- Stretches the spinal muscles, particularly in the lower back
- May relieve lower back pain and discomfort
- Induces overall relaxation

Downward Dog

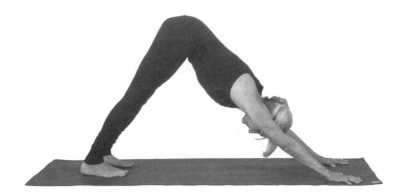

Description

1. Start on hands and knees with hands beneath the shoulders and knees slightly behind the hips. With straight arms and inner elbows facing each other, spread the fingers and palms, press the roots of the fingers firmly to the ground, and reach out through the fingertips.

2. Curl the toes under and press the hips up and back. Keep the legs bent to start, and actively press the hands into the floor while pressing the hips away from the hands and toward the ceiling.

3. Straighten the legs by pressing the thigh bones, shin bones, and heels back. Try to tilt the sitting bones toward the ceiling.

4. Contract the quadriceps while straightening the legs, but do not lock the knees.

5. Draw the belly in and widen the shoulder blades across the back.

6. The space between base of neck and upper arms (called the shoulder shelf) should be relaxed as the shoulder blades move toward the tailbone.

7. Let the head be heavy and relaxed.

Benefits

- Stretches the spinal muscles
- Rejuvenates the spinal discs
- Stretches the hamstrings, calves, Achilles tendon, arches, and hands
- Stretches the shoulders and chest
- Strengthens the wrists, arms, legs, and upper body
- Is an all-over rejuvenating stretch
- Is an absolute *must* pose for runners

Staff Pose

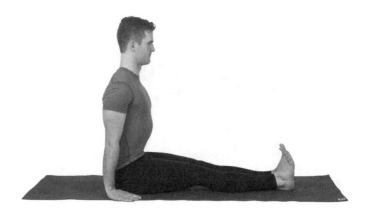

Description

1. In a seated position, clear flesh from the sitting bones so they are equally grounded.
2. Straighten the legs and roll the thighs inward slightly.
3. Flex the feet and push forward through the heels. Spread the toes and press forward through the big-toe joints and toward you with the baby-toe joints.
4. Press the palms to the floor by the hips, release the shoulder blades down the back, and press them into the body so the breastbone lifts and collarbones broaden. Squeeze the back of the arm pits together.
5. The sacrum should be perpendicular to the ground; pull in the belly and the front of the ribs so the lower back feels supported.
6. Lengthen the spine from the base of the sacrum to the crown of the head.
7. If the lower back rounds, sit up on a block.

Benefits

- Teaches proper spinal alignment while seated, improving posture
- Stretches back muscles, shoulders, and chest
- Stretches hamstrings and calves
- Strengthens the abdominals

Simple Seated Twist

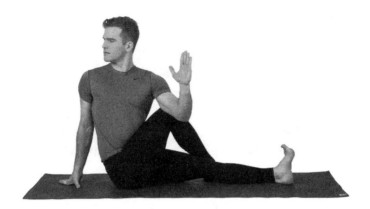

Description

1. From staff pose, bend the right leg and place the right foot outside the left thigh, keeping the right sitting bone grounded.

2. Wrap the left arm around the folded leg, and place the right hand on the floor behind you. For a deeper twist, the left elbow can be placed at the right outer knee with the hand in a stop-sign position. Press the arm and knee into each other to provide resistance.

3. Pressing the thigh toward the chest, rotate the torso to the right from the base of the spine, lengthening the spine as the twist deepens. Do not lean; rather, pull the sides of the torso in to keep the spine erect. Turn the head to softly gaze over the right shoulder.

4. Press the shoulder blades down the back. Lift the right side of the chest.

5. Hold the pose; with every inhale, lengthen the spine, and with every exhale, deepen the twist.

6. Unwind yourself and return to staff pose.

7. Repeat on the other side.

Benefits

- Stretches and tones the muscles of the back
- Stretches and strengthens the abdominal obliques
- Stimulates blood flow to the spinal vertebrae
- Improves flexibility of the spine
- Stimulates vital organs

Thighs to Chest

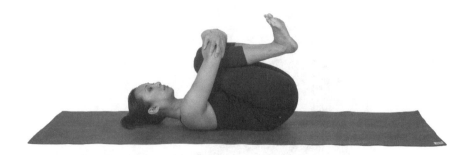

Description

1. Lying supine, bend the knees, wrap the arms around the shins, and press the thighs into the chest.
2. Flex the feet, soften the abdomen, and draw the knees closer to the chest. Breathe deeply and feel the lower back expand as it presses into the floor with the inhale.

Variations

1. Raise the head and bring the forehead to the knees for a deeper stretch.
2. Slowly roll from side to side for a lower-back massage.
3. Rock forward and back on the spine.
4. Make circles with the knees in one direction and then in the other.

Benefits

- Stretches the entire back, particularly the lower back
- Massages and mobilizes the spine
- Induces overall relaxation

Supine Twist

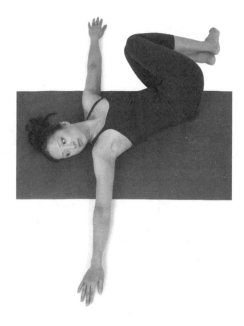

Description

1. From thighs to chest pose, extend the arms out to the sides, at shoulder height, with palms down. Keeping knees together, roll them to the left toward the left elbow and as close to the floor as possible.
2. Turn the head and gaze to the right.
3. Press the right shoulder toward the ground. Breathe deeply into the right ribs.
4. Repeat on the other side.

Benefits

- Stretches and tones the spinal muscles
- Mobilizes the spinal vertebrae
- Stretches the obliques and glutes

Chest Opener

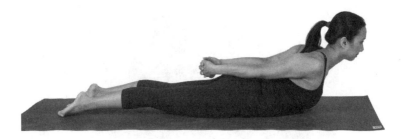

Description

1. Lie prone with the forehead resting on the floor and the tops of the feet pressing into the floor. Rotate outer ankles inward so they do not splay and tops of the feet are flat on the floor.
2. Interlace fingers behind the back.
3. Straighten and lift the arms away from the body, press the knuckles toward the feet, and lift the chest away from the floor. Pull the navel in toward the lower back.
4. Press the tops of the feet into the floor and energize the legs so the knees and lower thighs come off the ground.
5. Press the front hip bones into the floor.
6. Press the shoulder blades down the back to broaden the collar bones and open the chest.

Benefits

- Strengthens the spinal muscles
- Strengthens the hamstrings
- Strengthens the core
- Stretches the shoulders, chest, and abdominals
- Counteracts upper-back rounding and improves posture

Cobra

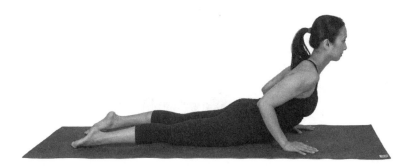

Description

1. Set up as in chest opener pose.
2. Bend the arms and place the hands by the lower ribs so that elbows are approximately over the wrists. Hug the elbows into the body and extend them toward the feet so you feel the shoulder blades slide down the back.
3. Spread the toes and press the tops of the feet into the floor, energizing the legs so that the knees and lower thighs begin to come off the ground.
4. Lengthen the sides of the torso forward and lift the chest, directing the sternum toward the ceiling. Slowly start to straighten the arms to further lift the chest off the floor, up to a height where the hips stay on the floor. Keep the elbows hugging the body and the front hip bones pressing into the floor.
5. Do not let the shoulders lift to the ears; rather, press them down the back and forward into the upper back to further expand the chest.
6. Gaze forward or slightly upward, being careful not to jut the chin forward and crunch the back of the neck. Keep the back of the neck long.

Benefits

- Strengthens the spinal muscles
- Strengthens the hamstrings
- Strengthens the core
- Stretches the shoulders, chest, and abdominals
- Counteracts upper-back rounding and improves posture

Locust

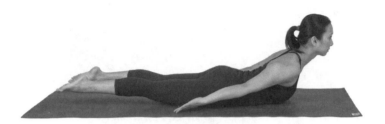

Description

1. Set up as for chest opener pose.
2. Arms are straight, by your side with palms up.
3. Press the front hip bones into the floor.
4. Press the tops of the hands into the floor, widen the collarbones, and lift the chest and upper body away from the floor, directing the sternum forward and toward the ceiling. Let the head lift, following the movement of the upper body and keep it in line with the shoulders. Contract the abdomen to support the lower back.
5. Straighten the legs and contract the hamstrings. Strongly press the tops of the feet into the floor and spread the toes. Keeping the front hip bones grounded, lift the legs off the floor from the tops of the thighs with no bend at the knee. Do not let the legs splay; keep them hip-distance apart. Strongly contract the muscles of the legs to keep them straight. If there is discomfort in the lower back, lift only one leg and repeat with the other leg.
6. Raise the arms parallel to the floor and reach through the fingertips. Imagine a weight pressing down on the backs of the upper arms, and push up toward the ceiling against this resistance. Press the shoulder blades firmly into the back and keep broadening the collarbones.
7. Gaze forward or slightly upward, being careful not to jut the chin forward and crunch the back of the neck. Keep the back of the neck long.

Benefits

- Strengthens the spinal muscles
- Strengthens the hamstrings
- Strengthens the core
- Stretches the shoulders, chest, and abdomen
- Counteracts upper-back rounding and improves posture

Savasana (Corpse Pose)

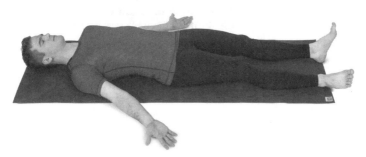

Description

1. Lie supine with legs outstretched, feet hip-distance apart, and arms at your sides with palms up. If the chin is higher than the forehead, place a folded blanket under the head.

2. If there is any discomfort in the lower back with the legs straight, place a bolster or rolled blanket beneath the knees. Alternatively, bend the legs and keep the knees together and the feet hip-distance apart.

3. Gently close your eyes. Roll the head from side to side as you soften and release any tension in the neck and shoulders. Let the head come to rest in neutral with the back of the head centered on the floor. Allow the body weight to completely sink into the floor. Keep the jaw, throat, and mouth relaxed. Remain still while consciously relaxing every muscle and joint in the body.

4. If your mind wanders, gently bring your attention back to your body and breath. Hold. Your duration in this pose can be 3 to 10 minutes. Generally, the duration is geared to the length of the yoga practice; the longer the practice, the longer the savasana. There is no right or wrong with this pose; remain in it for as long as you have time.

5. Do not skip this pose! Even if you have a short practice, take at least a couple of minutes in this pose.

6. To come out of the pose, slowly move the fingers, toes, wrists, and ankles; extend the arms overhead; and stretch out the legs and the arms. Slowly bend the knees and roll to one side, letting the head rest on the arm. Remain in this fetal position for a few moments, and then come up to seated. Pause for a moment of gratitude, observe the feelings and sensations in your body and mind; then be on your way!

Benefits

- Normalizes the body and helps the body integrate the benefits from the yoga practice
- Relaxes the body and mind
- Stimulates the parasympathetic nervous system, which heals and nourishes the body, as well as slows the heart rate and the breath. Leaves you feeling calm yet energized

REFERENCES

Sherman, K.J., D.C. Cherkin, R.D. Wellman, et al. 2011. A Randomized Trial Comparing Yoga, Stretching, and a Self-Care Book for Chronic Low Back Pain. *Archives of Internal Medicine* 171(22): 2019-2026. doi:10.1001/archinternmed.2011.524.

Chapter 8

Core Strength: Maximize Your Running Performance

When asked to define the core, until recently, most of us would have said the abdominals. But thanks to the increasing popularity of such disciplines as Pilates and yoga, the definition of the core has become more refined.

Everyone would agree that the core includes the abdominals, but we have broadened this definition to include a number of other muscle groups. For our purposes, we include many muscles of the torso, including the front, sides, and back of the body, as well as the pelvic floor and upper body. Note that some of the muscles that attach to the hips have a role in connecting the legs to the torso and determine core strength. These muscles are examined in chapter 10 (hips).

Along with more knowledge of what the core actually is, we also have more information about the relationship between core strength and athletic performance. In fact, pick up any fitness-related magazine, and you will be sure to find at least one article on core strengthening. Performance in virtually every sport can only benefit from having a strong core.

A strong core is also fundamental to good health, supporting virtually all of your daily movements. Whether you are sitting, standing, walking, ascending or descending stairs, running, twisting, or lifting objects, a strong core will ease the effort. And if you suffer from lower-back pain, the ubiquitous treatment plan involves core strengthening.

STRUCTURE OF THE CORE

Let's begin by examining the main muscle groups that encompass the core. Note that this is not intended to be a comprehensive examination of all related muscles, but rather the key ones that you should be alert to, to have a safe and highly effective yoga practice.

Abdominal Muscles

The abdominal muscles (figure 8.1) play a leading role in core strength. They include a group of muscles that collectively support the torso from the front, sides, and back, extending from the pelvis to the lower ribs. They support the body in movement while creating the stability to keep you upright. They are essential in postural support and have a role in breathing, especially during the exhalation, where they help expel the air from the lungs. Generally, the deeper in the body and closer to the spine the abdominal muscle is located, the more effectively it supports the torso and the spine in particular.

Rectus Abdominis   The rectus abdominis is the most superficial abdominal muscle and produces the six-pack look that has become the model to which many aspire. The role of the rectus abdominis is to flex, bend the spine forward, and bring the rib cage to the pelvis, as in a crunch. Because many seek the rippled six-pack definition, this muscle is often overworked. As with other muscles that are overly contracted, the rectus abdominis can become overly tight, shorten, and maintain the body in

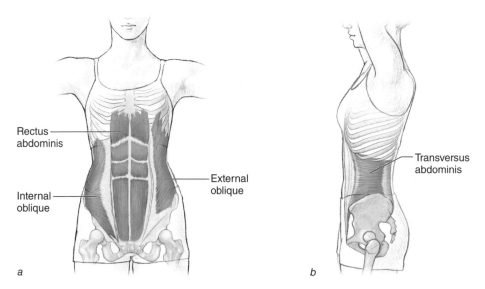

Rectus abdominis

Internal oblique

External oblique

Transversus abdominis

a

b

▶ **Figure 8.1**   The abdominal muscles.

a constant state of flexion. This has a detrimental effect on the natural curves of the spine.

That is not to say that the rectus abdominis muscle does not need to be strong. It does, but it also needs to be able to lengthen to extend the body, as in back bends. Furthermore, a strong and supple rectus abdominis supports the spine without altering its natural curves.

Obliques The obliques comprise two sets of muscles, the internal and external obliques. They are layered and thus provide tremendous postural support for the trunk. The muscle fibers of the internal and external obliques run in different directions and work synergistically to rotate the torso, allowing the trunk to twist and extend from side to side.

Transversus Abdominis (TA) The transversus abdominis, or TA, the deepest of the abdominal muscles, wraps around the body much like a corset. It plays a crucial role in supporting the spine and stabilizing the lumbar spine and pelvis while flattening the abdominal wall and holding the internal organs in place. It is considered a key muscle in core stability. Unlike the other abdominal muscles, the TA is less obvious and thus often overlooked in workouts. It engages autonomically in bodily functions such as coughing, vomiting, and childbirth. Learning to isolate and contract the TA while stationary and in movement is vital to weight-bearing yoga poses, such as arm balances and chaturanga (yoga push-up). Although at first, engaging the TA is a conscious action, eventually it becomes automatic and is a great way to work core strength into your *Yoga for Runners* practice.

Unlike other muscles that shorten and lead to misalignment elsewhere in the body, the TA simply becomes stronger the more it is worked. A strong and healthy TA braces the body and stabilizes the torso so that other muscles can work effectively. If you are interested in running strong and efficiently and reducing the risk of injury, you must include specific core-strengthening work, especially by finding and working the TA.

FINDING THE TRANSVERSUS ABDOMINIS

Depending on how they are done, traditional abdominal crunches may or may not strengthen the TA. If this muscle is weak, the work naturally transfers to the rectus abdominis, obliques, or hip flexors. Given the vital role of the TA, it is important to learn how to engage and strengthen it. As you become familiar with the actions of this muscle, it will become stronger, and engaging it through various movements and exercises will become second nature. At the outset, however, you need to learn to isolate and feel this muscle.

1. Lie supine with legs bent, feet hip-distance apart, and arms comfortably resting by your sides.

2. To place the pelvis in neutral, press the feet into the floor, lift the pelvis a few inches off the floor, and slowly release it to the floor. The sacrum should lie flat on the floor.

3. The spine should be in neutral, and the lumbar spine curve should leave a small space between the floor and the back. However, if the neutral spine produces a larger arch or no arch at all, do not purposely alter it. Your body will naturally go to its own version of neutral at the outset. As your yoga practice improves muscle imbalances, the spinal curves will change.

4. Take a few deep abdominal breaths (see chapter 3), softening and relaxing the belly from the outside and deeply to the inside.

5. Place your fingertips at the two protruding hip bones at the front of the pelvis. Slide your fingertips inward about 1 to 2 inches (2.5 to 5 cm), toward the center of the belly. Keeping the pelvis still, cough a few times and feel the muscle contraction beneath your fingertips. This is the transversus abdominis. Cough a few times and observe how this muscle contracts and flattens the belly without altering the lower-back arch.

6. Now consciously contract the TA to produce the same effect as when coughing. You should feel the lower abdomen flatten, creating a hollowness. Imagine a corset pulling in the abdomen as the laces are pulled and tightened. Do not let the pelvis tilt or the lower ribs flare upward.

7. Hold this contraction for five deep ujjayi breaths (see chapter 3); then release. Be sure to relax the shoulders, neck, and jaw.

8. Repeat 5 to 10 times.

It is easiest to start the TA isolation and contraction work while in a supine position. Once you are able to create this abdominal hollowing, you can do it in any position. Note that while standing, it is particularly important that the lower ribs not flare upward. This is a very effective way to brace the spine and is useful when carrying and lifting objects, rising from a chair, or bending forward. Also, keep it in mind if you feel your posture sagging during your run.

Iliopsoas

The psoas is tubular in shape and forms part of the iliopsoas (figure 8.2), which includes the psoas major, psoas minor, and the iliacus. The psoas attaches to T12 and all the lumbar vertebrae, meets the iliacus at the hip, and forms one tendon that inserts at the inner femur. The iliopsoas is rather elusive; it is the deepest core muscle and the only one that directly connects the spine to the leg. It is key in the health of the spine.

Because the iliopsoas is so deep in the body and we can't feel or see it, many people are unaware that they even have it. Yet it plays such a vital role in both core strength and spinal health that you should become familiar with its workings. You take an average of 2,000 to 2,500 steps in every mile, and as the strongest of the hip flexors, the iliopsoas contracts with every step. In addition, the iliopsoas is in a constant state of contraction while seated; most of us spend a considerable amount of

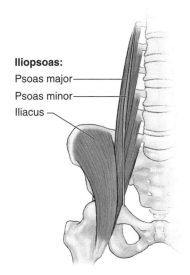

Iliopsoas:
Psoas major—
Psoas minor—
Iliacus—

▶ **Figure 8.2** The iliopsoas.

time seated throughout our lives and very little time, if any, stretching it. Thus, you can see why it is so tight for many of us.

The iliopsoas stabilizes the pelvis and midsection, as well as the abdominals and lower-back muscles. Greater stability in this area permits the legs to move with greater ease and efficiency. Therefore, the function of the iliopsoas is especially important for runners. With every stride, the iliopsoas is in use, contracting when the front leg pushes forward and lengthening as the leg extends back. A healthy iliopsoas accommodates this movement by contracting and lengthening at the appropriate times, contributing to a long and fluid stride, whereas a tight iliopsoas leads to a short and choppy stride, or shuffle. Many of us mostly ignore the iliopsoas in our workouts, especially when stretching. However, a number of yoga poses call on the iliopsoas to either contract to create stability or to stretch, providing the opportunity to lengthen it.

A healthy iliopsoas also works smoothly with other muscles to support an upright posture. A short iliopsoas leads to spinal misalignment and poor posture by increasing the arch of the lower back and tilting the pelvis forward. If this is the pattern in your body, it will likely become your posture while running, which can cause a host of misalignment issues in the hips, knees, or lower back. In addition, a tight iliopsoas creates pressure in the lower back, leading to lower-back pain and compression of the lumbar discs.

Pelvic Floor

For a complete picture of core strength, we need to examine the pelvic floor (figure 8.3). For most of us, this is a truly esoteric part of the body and not typically part of our workouts. Yet in yoga, contracting the pelvic floor is considered a fundamental component of core strength; this practice is known as mula bandha, or root lock.

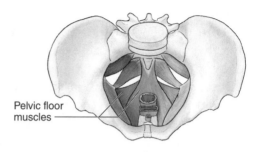

▶ **Figure 8.3** The pelvic floor.

The pelvic floor, also called the pelvic diaphragm, is made up of several muscles at the base of the torso and is situated between the two sitting bones, the tailbone, and the pubic bone. The pelvic floor may be overly tight or overly weak and, like any muscle in the body, needs toning. Imagine this layer of muscles as a trampoline that rises when contracted and releases when relaxed. During yoga practice, you should learn to consciously contract the pelvic floor when needed while at other times stretching it out. The result is a healthy and toned pelvic floor that provides a host of health benefits.

A toned pelvic floor provides support for the bladder, intestines, rectum, and uterus. Furthermore, these muscles work with the abdominal and back muscles to stabilize and support the spine. Commonly, pelvic floor exercises, known as Kegel exercises, are undertaken during pregnancy and often forgotten soon after. A weakened pelvic floor can result in pain in the lower back and pelvic area.

Once you are familiar with contracting the pelvic floor, you can do it anywhere and at any time to strengthen it, but it is important to integrate this work into your yoga practice. In yoga, mula bandha is considered helpful for containing the flow of energy; it is used in various breathing techniques to increase energy and vitality. Using this root lock with physical postures increases core strength and helps with more dynamic yoga sequences that involve jumping forward or back, inducing a feeling of lightness in the movement.

Engaging the pelvic floor also supports the body from the base of the core, allowing the arms and legs to be more relaxed in poses while enabling longer holds in poses with less effort. In addition, mula bandha stabilizes the pelvis, protecting the lower back and sacrum from strain and overstretching.

FINDING THE PELVIC FLOOR

Stretching the pelvic floor is relatively easy and done naturally in a number of yoga poses where the legs are widely spread. Strengthening the pelvic floor requires a more concentrated effort. This simple isometric exercise, done in isolation, will begin your journey of strengthening the pelvic floor. Note that as this work becomes easier, the contraction and relaxation is included throughout the yoga practice, seamlessly integrating the energetic and physical body. Initially, this exercise may be frustrating because you may not feel anything. Don't give up! This work is as subtle as it is powerful.

1. Lie supine in a comfortable position with legs bent. The head can be supported with a folded blanket if needed.

2. Take a few long deep breaths, inhaling and exhaling deeply (see chapter 3).

3. Draw your attention to your pelvic floor, the layer of muscles between the sitting bones, pubic bone, and tailbone.

4. Exhale and consciously contract this layer of muscles, pulling them upward and inward; hold for 5 to 10 seconds. It may be helpful to visualize a spiraling flow of energy rising upward through the center of the body. You will also feel the lower deep abdominal muscles contract. Do not tilt the pelvis, and do not contract the buttocks or thighs.

5. Inhale and completely relax the pelvic floor muscles.

6. Repeat contracting and releasing for five breaths. Take a few relaxed abdominal breaths.

7. Repeat the cycle three to five times.

It is important to coordinate the contraction and relaxation with your breathing. At first, you may need to exert a bit of effort to feel the contraction, even overcontracting just to feel something. Over time, however, the effort will reduce as your body is able to feel the subtle sensations of this work. As you become more proficient with this exercise, you will be able to do it while seated or standing. This is a great exercise to do while standing and waiting in line or even while sitting in a car. Experiment with it and use it as a source of energy when needed, as when running up a hill or skipping up the stairs.

• •

Upper Body

The muscles of the upper body are also a vital component of core strength (figure 8.4). We will specifically examine those muscles that we must be aware of in a strengthening type of yoga practice, such as the *Yoga for Runners* sequences. Although we will not be specifically examining the arm muscles, the work done to strengthen the upper body also strengthens the arms, including the upper arms, wrists, and hands.

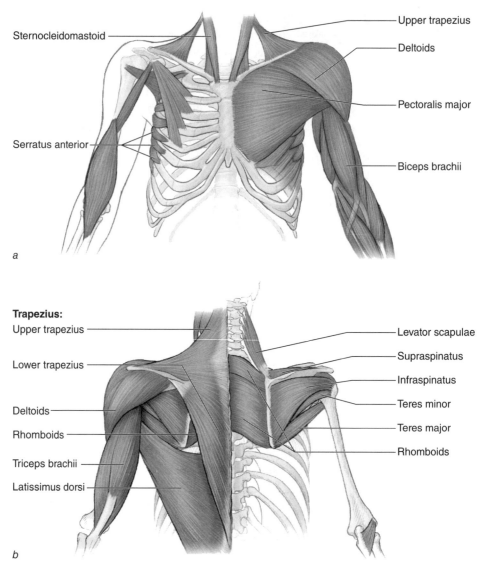

Figure 8.4 The upper body: *(a)* front view and *(b)* back view.

Although running exercises the lower body, the upper body is not strengthened, leaving many runners weak in this area. Yet if you seek a balance of strength, flexibility, and endurance, upper-body strength is indispensable. Examine any runner, and it is easy to see that the upper body is an integral part of the stride. Although not directly bearing weight, the arms are in motion to counterbalance the movement of the legs and propel the body forward. By our definition, upper-body strength is a component of core strength, and a strong upper body helps maintain postural alignment and form, providing vital support to the body so it can run efficiently and with speed.

A great deal of emphasis is placed on the upper body in the *Yoga for Runners* program. The first and perhaps most vital thing that yoga teaches is body awareness. You learn and continually practice how to pull the shoulders down the back, broaden the collarbones to open the chest, and stand tall, which is helpful alignment in all aspects of your life, whether in movement or while sedentary. Let's take a quick look at the key muscles to be aware of in your yoga practice.

Trapezius The trapezius is a diamond-shaped muscle that is situated along the thoracic spine. The upper trapezius attaches to the outside of the shoulder blade, so contracting it lifts the shoulders, as in shrugging. This muscle is often in a state of constant contraction through lifestyle tendencies such as carrying the head forward from its neutral position, holding a phone between the head and shoulders, carrying heavy purses or bags, and overall poor posture. It also tightens when we hunch, especially when we are under stress. Chronic tightness in this area is very common. The lower trapezius contracts to draw the shoulder blades down the back and stabilizes the shoulders, which is especially important when weight bearing. A typical condition is for the upper trapezius to be overly tight and the lower trapezius to be weak. This contributes to the condition of a rounded upper back and a shortening of the neck. Runners commonly complain of shoulder and neck tension during and after runs. If your typical posture includes tight upper traps and hunched shoulders, this is the posture you will assume while running, and the condition will only worsen through the run. In addition to being a nuisance and the cause of discomfort, this tightness is a drain on your energy and leaves you more susceptible to fatigue.

The first step to relieving the stress and strain in the neck and shoulders is to develop body awareness. It is often one of the lessons students learn in their first yoga classes. From this heightened awareness, you learn to be more attentive to this key aspect of posture when sitting, standing, walking, and running, continually reinforcing drawing the shoulder blades down the back and keeping the head over the shoulders. Furthermore, practicing some simple stretch techniques can give instant relief, and treatments such as massage therapy and using a hard ball to roll out tight spots can offer temporary relief.

The long-term fix is to strengthen the muscles of the upper body, a key one being the lower trapezius. A strong lower trapezius will counteract the effect of the overly tight upper trapezius, and upper body carriage will improve while the nagging neck and shoulder tension subsides. Yoga poses that bear body weight require that the lower trapezius muscle be engaged. At the beginning, many of these poses are challenging, but when mindfully executed with proper attention to detail and alignment, these supportive muscles will strengthen to create balanced and useful upper-body strength for daily activities.

Serratus Anterior The serratus anterior is a little more obscure than the other muscles of the upper body because it isn't readily visible, yet it is of prime importance in supporting the upper torso and in upper-body movement. When contracted, it holds the shoulder blade in place and stabilizes the shoulder joint, as when pressing the arms against resistance in a yoga push-up (chaturanga).

The serratus anterior is used in many yoga poses and is key to proper form. When the arms are raised, the serratus anterior works to keep the shoulder blades down. As with the lower trapezius, strengthening this muscle reduces upper-body tension while preventing the shoulders from climbing to the ears. In addition, the serratus anterior is fundamental in weight-bearing yoga poses, providing upper-body strength and stability to enable you to safely execute challenging poses.

Latissimus Dorsi Latissimus dorsi literally means "broadest muscle of the back." Like other muscles, for optimum function, it needs to have strength and flexibility. When this muscle is tight, it compresses the back and restricts the range of motion of the arm, which can compress the shoulder joint and lead to rotator cuff injury. When lifting heavy objects, the latissimus dorsi helps stabilize the arm bone in the shoulder joint.

The latissimus dorsi, along with the other superficial and deep muscles of the back, are stretched in many yoga poses, the most basic one being extending the arms straight overhead while keeping the arm bones in their sockets. Additionally, these muscles are strengthened in the back-bending family of poses. This blend of strength and flexibility is what contributes to a strong back, improved posture, and a strong torso to support the weight-bearing action of running with ease.

RUNNING, YOGA, AND CORE STRENGTH

As promoted in disciplines such as yoga, Pilates, dance, and martial arts, core strength is the key component to moving efficiently and safely, and with grace and poise. The core is the center from which the legs and arms move. It is the body's power hub and needs to be strong for stability and flexible to permit movement. Regardless of the sport, a strong core is a must for optimum athletic performance.

One of the first times you made the connection between your core and athletics may have been when you learned to throw a ball. Rather than throwing the ball from the arm, you may have been encouraged to put your weight behind the ball for greater power and longer distance. Examining the actions related to running, the moving parts are the legs and, to a lesser degree, the arms. However, the power behind the movement comes from the core. A strong core stabilizes the torso, eliminates unnecessary movements, and allows the legs and arms to move with greater efficiency and ease. In essence, a strong core supports the movement of the legs and creates a lightness so they can more easily propel the body forward.

More efficiency in the running stride results in less fatigue, greater endurance, fewer injuries, faster running times, and happier runners. A strong core is essential for strong running. A strong core does the following:

- Supports the torso during the weight-bearing action of running
- Supports the movement of the legs, giving them lightness so they can more easily propel you forward
- Supports the spine and the delicate central nervous system
- Improves posture, supporting a more upright body carriage to improve spinal alignment and overall body alignment
- Increases confidence and self-esteem through improved posture
- Increases endurance because there is less energy drain on the body and less fatigue, which is especially important during longer runs
- Improves functional movement, including bending, twisting, lifting, walking, climbing, and running
- Strengthens the back, prevents back injuries, and reduces the risk of injury when lifting objects
- Improves balance and stability

Many people are under the misconception that yoga is strictly for flexibility. Although improving flexibility is a key benefit of yoga, there is also tremendous strengthening to be gained, which is an essential requirement for creating a balanced and healthy body. A balanced yoga practice requires the body to move in all planes—front and back, side to side, rotation, and even upside down. Yoga requires the body to move in an integrated way, much as you do during your natural movements throughout the day—for example, bending forward to pick something up, looking over your shoulder when making a lane change, twisting the body to pick up something in the back seat, reaching the arms overhead to grab something from a high shelf, and carrying heavy objects. In all of these relatively simple movements, the core has a function.

Truly beneficial core strengthening uses many muscles to coordinate the movement. Unlike weightlifting, in which a muscle or joint is worked in isolation, core strength in yoga is an integrated approach combining strength, flexibility, and often balance. Many muscle groups work at the same time, some contracting and some stretching, to perform their function in supporting the pose. Depending on the pose, this can include the muscles of the abdominals, back, shoulders, chest, arms, and legs. Your own body weight provides the weight-bearing component. How simple is that?

Headstands are an excellent example of the entire body working in an integrated fashion to produce stability. Contrary to what the name of the pose implies, only 30 to 40 percent of the weight is on the head. The remainder of the weight is held through the torso, and the arms serve as the bridge between the ground and the trunk. Rather than adding to the weight, the legs strongly extend upward to help reduce the effect of gravity and do their part in reducing the weight on the head.

A stable headstand requires a blend of strength, flexibility, and balance, but chiefly a strong and stable core. When students learn the headstand, they often comment on how much abdominal strength is required to first lift the legs and then hold the body upright. Although this is true, the muscles of the neck, shoulders, arms, and back, along with the hip stabilizers, are also very engaged to create the needed stability. Amazingly, once the body is in alignment, stable, and balanced, it is virtually effortless to be upside down. The body works as an integrated unit, combining strength with ease so you can hold the pose for several minutes.

Core strength work in yoga is integrated into every pose. That is, every pose requires you to be centered, balanced, and stable. For example, when you bend forward, you pull in the navel to support the lower back; in standing poses, you move from the center and support the spine; and in back bends, you contract and strengthen the back muscles while stretching the front of the body. There are also poses that more specifically isolate muscle groups, as detailed in this chapter and in the yoga sequences in chapter 12.

Just as the muscles of the upper body and core support the spine when you are upside down, as in a headstand, these same muscles serve us well when you are on your feet. They stabilize the torso, support your upright body carriage, improve posture, and facilitate all functional movements, including running.

YOGA POSES FOR THE CORE

The poses described in this section are for strengthening the core, as defined in this chapter. When doing challenging work, contract the pelvic floor for added strength and stability. Some of these poses are to simply stretch out the pesky neck and shoulders that so often come under duress.

Ab Curls I

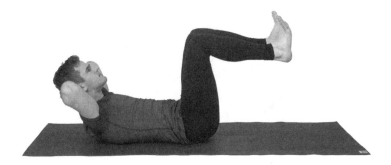

Description

1. Lie supine with legs bent and feet hip-distance apart.

2. Press the feet into the floor, lift the pelvis a few inches off the ground, and slowly release it to the floor. The sacrum lies flat on the floor, and the spine is in neutral.

3. Hollow the belly by pulling the navel toward the lower back, but do not tilt the pelvis. Contract the transversus abdominis as described previously in this chapter.

4. Lift the feet off the ground, with the knees over the hips and the shins parallel to the floor. Flex the feet.

5. Interlace the fingers behind the head and curl the chest, shoulders, and head off the floor. Let the head fall completely heavy into the hands.

6. With a hollow belly, inhale into the lower back, and on the exhale, lift the upper body a bit more. Note that the movement will be small, yet controlled.

7. Throughout this exercise, do *not* do the following:
   - Release the head and shoulders to the floor between curls
   - Use momentum
   - Jerk the upper body toward the legs
   - Let the legs move toward the upper body
   - Let the hips move from side to side
   - Tighten the neck and jaw

Benefit

- Strengthens the transversus abdominis

Ab Curls II

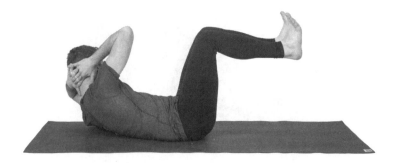

Description

1. Perform the action as described in ab curls I, but on each exhale, reach the elbow to the opposite knee.

2. Keeping the head and chest lifted, return to center on the inhale and exhale to the other side.

Note: Avoid the actions listed in step 7 of the description of ab curls I. Also, when extending the elbow, lift the shoulder and upper back from the floor; do not move the knee toward the elbow.

Benefit

- Strengthens and stretches the obliques

Plank

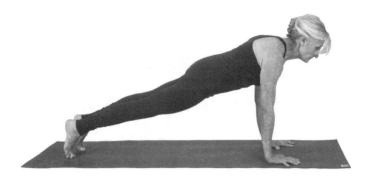

Description

1. From hands and knees, spread the fingers and press the bases of the index fingers into the floor. Hands are shoulder-distance apart, and knees and feet are hip-distance apart.
2. Keeping the shoulders over the wrists, step the feet back until the body is parallel to the floor.
3. Pull the upper arm bones back to secure the shoulder joint.
4. Firm the shoulder blades against the back and spread them away from the spine.
5. Spread the collarbones and lift the breastbone.
6. Press back through the heels and contract the thighs.
7. Hollow the belly and lift the lower ribs. Press the tailbone toward the heels. The body is on one plane from head to feet.
8. Look up slightly, keeping the throat and eyes soft.
9. Throughout this exercise and the next (chaturanga), do *not* do the following:
   - Let the pelvis or belly sink.
   - Let the head drop.
   - Let the shoulders move toward the ears.
   - Let the elbows splay from the body.
   - Let the upper arm bones tilt toward floor.

Benefits

- Strengthens the upper body, shoulders, and chest
- Strengthens arms and wrists
- Strengthens the legs
- Strengthens the abdominals

Chaturanga (Yoga Push-Up)

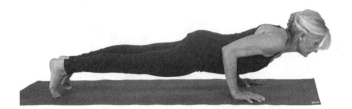

Description

1. From plank, shift your weight forward and slowly lower the body toward the floor until the upper arms are parallel to the floor with the elbows over the wrists.

2. Pause and then lower the body to the ground, trying to keep the arms at 90 degrees.

3. Keep the elbows in; they should brush the sides of the body on the way down.

4. Keep the shoulder blades pressing into the back and the collarbones broad.

5. Keep the head in line with the shoulders.

6. After bringing the body to the floor, extend the toes so the tops of the feet rest on the floor.

7. From the floor, you can either move into upward dog, as in the sun salutation sequence, or you can press the hands into the floor, lift the entire torso until the arms are straight, and press the hips back into downward dog.

Benefits

- Works the entire core
- Strengthens the abdominals, shoulders, upper back, chest, arms, and wrists
- Stretches the soles of the feet
- Strengthens the legs

Side Plank

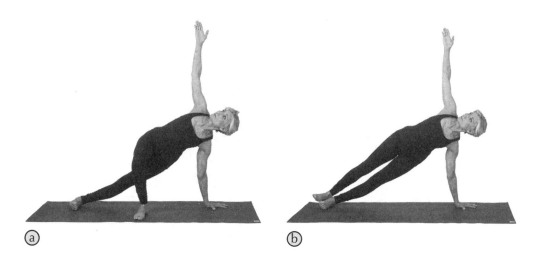

(a)   (b)

Description

1. From plank, bring the feet together and turn to one side by pivoting on the toes so that the outer edge of the bottom foot rests on the floor. Top leg position variations include:
   - The top leg bent (as in a kickstand, *a*),
   - feet side by side, top foot resting on inner edge,
   - feet stacked *(b)*, or
   - top leg lifted.
2. Stack the hips and shoulders and lift the bottom hip so there is no sagging.
3. Position the supporting hand beneath the shoulder and firmly press the shoulder away from the ear. Straighten the arm by firming the triceps, and press the base of the index finger firmly into the floor.
4. Extend the top arm toward the ceiling, in line with the shoulders.
5. Squeeze the inner thighs and press out through the soles of the feet.
6. Align the entire body into one line from the feet to the crown of the head.
7. Keep the head aligned with the shoulders, and gently turn your gaze to the extended hand.
8. Hold for desired number of breaths; pivot on the feet to return to all fours, and then pivot to the other side.

Benefits

- Works the entire core
- Strengthens the abdominals, shoulders, upper back, chest, arms, legs, ankles, and wrists

Dolphin (Downward Dog Variation)

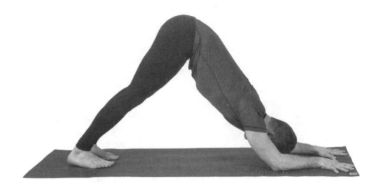

Description

1. From downward dog (chapter 7), release the knees to the floor. Place the forearms and hands (fingers spread) on the floor, align the elbows beneath the shoulders, and keep the forearms parallel and the wrists in line with the elbows.

2. Press your weight through the length of the forearms to the extended fingers, and press the inner wrists to the floor.

3. Strongly press the upper arm bones toward the legs, lift the shoulder blades away from the ears, and press them into the back.

4. Draw the navel in, curl the toes under, and straighten the legs, coming into a downward dog variation.

5. Let the head fall between the upper arms; do not rest it on the floor.

6. Press the hips away from the hands, and strongly press the upper thighs, shin bones, and heels back.

7. Continue to press the upper arm bones toward the legs, and the shoulder blades away from the ears.

Benefits

- Strengthens the upper body
- Strengthens the arms and legs
- Strengthens the abdominals
- Stretches the spine
- Stretches the shoulders, hamstrings, calves, and arches

Dolphin Plank

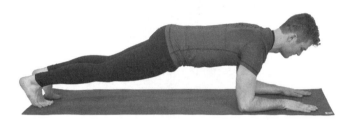

Description

1. From dolphin, walk the feet back and drop the hips so they are in line with the upper body.
2. Press your weight through the length of the forearms to the extended fingers, and roll the inner wrists to the floor.
3. Strongly pull in the belly and front ribs.
4. Do not lift the hips; let the full weight of the sacrum settle into the pelvis.
5. Press the upper arms toward the legs, and press the shoulder blades away from the ears and into the back.

Benefits

- Strengthens the chest, upper body, and abdominals
- Stretches the shoulders, toes, and soles of the feet

Upward Plank

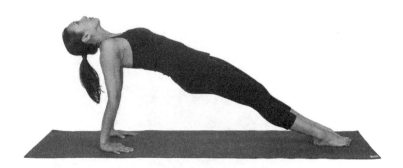

Description

1. Sit in staff pose (chapter 7) and place the hands about 6 to 8 inches (15 to 20 cm) behind the hips, with the fingers pointing forward.

2. With straight arms, press into the hands, curl the tailbone under, lift the hips, and straighten the legs. Point the toes.

3. Ensure that the wrists are under the shoulder joints.

4. Press the shoulder blades against the back and lift the chest.

5. Strongly contract the inner thighs and roll them inward. Extend the toes toward the floor, keeping the inner edges of the big toes together.

6. The head can softly release back, but do not fold the back of the neck. If this creates strain in the neck, keep the head in line with the shoulders.

Benefits

- Strengthens the arms, wrists, and legs
- Strengthens the back of the body
- Strengthens the legs
- Stretches the chest, shins, and ankles

Upward Dog

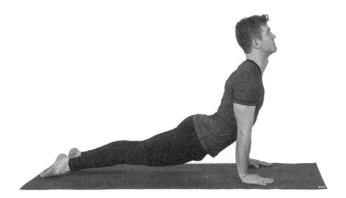

Description

1. Set up as in cobra (chapter 7).
2. Lie prone with the hands at the lower ribs so the elbows are over the wrists and the arms are at 90 degrees. Hug the elbows into the body and press them toward the feet.
3. Press the tops of the feet into the floor, energizing the legs so that the knees and lower thighs come off the ground.
4. Lift the head, keeping the muscles at the back of the neck relaxed. Press the hands into the floor, and slide the chest and upper torso forward through the arms until they straighten. The inner elbows are facing each other.
5. Continue lifting the chest, press into the tops of the feet, and straighten the legs.
6. Keep the shoulder blades away from the ears and press them against the back. Press the upper arm bones back to widen the collarbones while lifting the breastbone.
7. The thighs are firm, slightly rolled inward, and off the floor.
8. Letting the hips be heavy, lift the front hip bones toward the chest. Draw the belly in.
9. Look straight ahead or let the head gently fall back, but do not compress the back of the neck.

Benefits

- Strengthens and mobilizes the spine
- Strengthens the back muscles, arms, and wrists
- Stretches the chest, shoulders, and abdomen
- Stretches the hip flexors, ankles, and shins

Boat

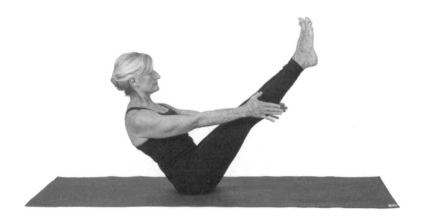

Description

1. Start in staff pose (chapter 7).
2. Bend the legs with the feet flat on the floor. Hollow the belly and move the thighs toward the chest.
3. Lift the breastbone and lean back slightly, remaining on the sitting bones.
4. Lift the feet from the floor and extend the legs until the calves are parallel to the floor.
5. Stretch the arms alongside the legs and reach strongly out through the fingers.
6. Press the shoulder blades into the back. If able to keep the belly hollow, straighten the legs until they are at a 45 degree angle.
7. Point the feet and spread the toes.
8. Gaze toward the feet.

Benefits

- Strengthens the abdominals
- Strengthens the spinal muscles
- Strengthens the psoas

Bridge

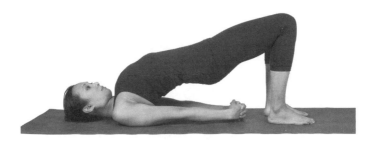

Description

1. Lie supine with legs bent, feet hip-distance apart, ankles beneath the knees, and toes pointed forward.
2. Press the inner feet and arms actively into the floor and, without tilting the pelvis, lift the hips and buttocks off the floor. Keep the thighs and inner feet parallel. Interlace the fingers below the hips and extend the hands toward the feet. Let the weight rest at the very top of the shoulders.
3. Press the backs of the upper arms to the floor, and lift the hips as high as possible.
4. Lift the chin slightly away from the breastbone, press the shoulder blades into the back, and lift the breastbone toward the chin.
5. Contract the hamstrings and inner thighs to keep the knees aligned over the ankles.
6. To come out of the pose, press the tailbone forward and drop the breastbone, upper back, lower back, and then the hips to the floor.

Benefits

- Strengthens the back muscles
- Strengthens the spine
- Strengthens the inner thighs
- Stretches the hip flexors
- Stretches the chest

Ear to Shoulder

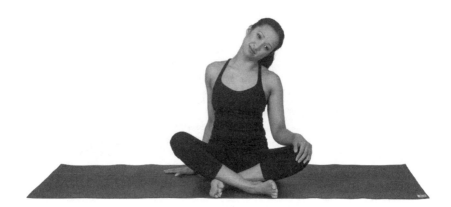

Description

1. Sit in staff pose (chapter 7) and cross the legs.
2. Rest the left hand on the knee and the right hand on the floor by the right hip.
3. Gradually let the head drop to the left ear, allowing the weight of the head to create the stretch. Press the right hand into the floor and press the right shoulder down to deepen the stretch.
4. Change the cross of the legs and the position of the arms and repeat on the other side.

Benefits

- Stretches the neck and upper trapezius
- Eases upper-body tightness

Cow Pose, Shoulder Stretch

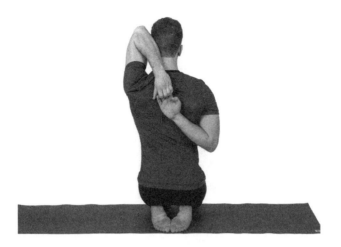

Description

1. Sitting in hero pose (chapter 6), place a belt (optional) over the left shoulder.
2. Extend the left arm up and drop the hand down the upper back. Keep the elbow in line with the shoulder joint and strongly reach it upward to stretch the entire left side of the body. Stretch the right arm to the right, in line with the shoulder joint and parallel to the floor. From the shoulder joint, rotate the arm inward (so the palm of the hand faces back and the thumb is pointing down); sweep the arm down and behind the torso.
3. Reach the hands toward each other. If they touch, clasp them together; otherwise, move them toward each other along the strap. Continue reaching the left elbow to the ceiling to deepen the stretch.
4. Keep the head upright in line with the shoulders.
5. Repeat on the other side.

Variation

1. This shoulder stretch can be done while standing also.

Benefits

- Stretches the side, armpits, triceps, and chest
- Releases shoulder and neck tension
- Increases range of motion in the shoulder joints

Eagle Arms

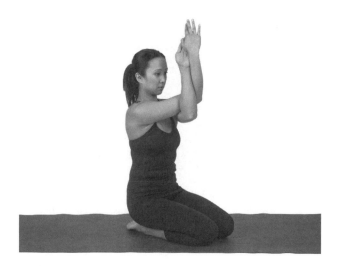

Description

1. Sit in staff pose (chapter 7) and cross the legs, or sit in hero pose (chapter 6).

2. Stretch the arms straight forward, parallel to the floor, and spread the shoulder blades wide across the upper back. Cross the arms in front of the torso so the right arm is above the left; then bend the elbows. Place the right elbow into the crook of the left elbow, and raise the forearms perpendicular to the floor.

3. The backs of the hands will be facing each other. If possible, interlace the forearms so the palms of the hands touch.

4. Press the palms together, lift the elbows so they are in line with the shoulders, and reach the fingers toward the ceiling.

5. Press the shoulder blades away from the ears.

6. Change the cross of the legs and repeat on the other side.

7. This pose can also be done while in equal standing.

Benefits

- Stretches the shoulders and upper back
- Releases shoulder and neck tension

Chapter 9

Hamstrings: Establish a Longer, More Fluid Stride

Tight hamstrings are the bane of existence for runners. A common sight at races is runners at the side of the road trying to unkink a knot in their hamstrings or limping along because they have literally become hamstrung.

Because tight hamstrings and running have come to be considered synonymous, runners are often surprised to learn that their hamstrings need to be stronger. Considering that the hamstrings repeatedly contract and extend with the running stride, the overall health and balance of this muscle group is of vital importance. This chapter explores the structure of the hamstrings, provides the many reasons for tight and weak hamstrings, and details yoga poses that can improve your hamstrings' overall health in order to add longevity to your running.

STRUCTURE OF THE HAMSTRINGS

Without the hamstrings, there would be no movement. They are involved in every step—walking, running, climbing, and even standing from a seated position. The functions of the hamstrings are fairly simple—to pull the leg back as the hip extends forward and to flex or bend the knee. The motion of running involves both of these actions on a continuous basis.

The hamstrings are the muscle mass at the back of upper leg, originating at the sitting bones and attaching at the lower leg bones (figure 9.1). The tightness felt at the back of the legs, especially when bending forward, is the hamstrings. The ubiquitous flexibility standard of touching your toes

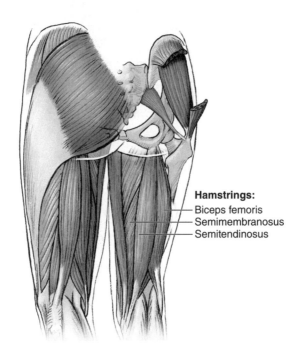

Hamstrings:
Biceps femoris
Semimembranosus
Semitendinosus

▶ **Figure 9.1** The hamstrings.

is largely a test of hamstring length. Tight hamstrings can have considerable impact on your freedom of movement and the health of your joints. Hamstrings are involved in many daily activities. How many times a day do you bend forward to pick something up or tie your shoelaces? It is very important to maintain a reasonable range of motion in the hamstrings to be able to move freely, safely, and painlessly.

Given the repetitive nature of running and the role of the hamstrings in every stride, it's no wonder that runners develop tight hamstrings. Tight hamstrings are a major cause of injury for runners, ranging from pain to strain to more debilitating muscle tears. As a result of being tight, the hamstrings become shorter at rest, which over time will shorten your running stride. Furthermore, tight hamstrings can alter hip balance, knee stability, and spinal alignment.

Tight hamstrings are not limited to runners, nor is running the only cause of tight hamstrings. While seated, the hamstring muscles are inactive and are held at a shortened length. Therefore, the tightening of the hamstrings starts at the age of five or six, when children begin their seated school careers. For many, this continues through the school years and into careers that require hours of sitting. Like other parts of the body, the hamstrings are adversely affected by sitting for extended periods of time.

Tight hamstrings can affect postural alignment. As discussed in chapter 7, neutral spinal alignment is required for optimal balance, symmetry, and effective weight bearing. When the resting length of the hamstrings shortens, a downward pull is exerted on the sitting bones, creating a rotation of the pelvis known as a posterior tilt. A posterior tilt in the pelvis can lead to hip problems, such as a strain on the sacroiliac joints. There is a strong interplay between the hamstrings and the hips, so the range of motion of the hip joint is also affected by tight hamstrings. A posterior tilt in the pelvis also flattens the precious lumbar curve and can lead to back problems, ranging from mild to severe back pain. In addition, a tucked pelvis creates imbalances in other sections of the spine, most notably rounded shoulders and a slouched posture while sitting, standing, or running.

Tight hamstrings also contribute to knee pain or injury. Because the hamstrings attach below the knee, their tightness can affect the knee joint, limiting the ability to fully straighten the leg. This affects the alignment of the knee joint, causing it to become compressed, and can contribute to knee pain or injury.

Shortened hamstrings will eventually reduce the length of your stride. Strong and supple hamstrings are necessary for a long, fluid, and unrestricted stride, allowing you to gain endurance and speed with less fatigue. With tight hamstrings, however, the ability to take long and fluid strides will be hindered and running efficiency and speed will be lost.

Finally, functionally tight hamstrings limit the hips' ability to hinge forward. If the hips do not move in forward bending, the spine will round instead and place a strain on the lumbar spine. A far too common lower-back injury occurs from the simple action of bending forward to pick up an object. The heavier the object is, the higher the likelihood of strain will be, but it can also occur when picking up something light, such as a pair of socks. The effect can be a muscle spasm, a strain, or a more severe herniation of a vertebral disk. Considering that on any given day you bend over numerous times for simple tasks, restoring length and strength to the hamstrings is a must for both your athletic performance and your overall health and well-being.

For runners, tight hamstrings pose a constant threat of discomfort and injury. Although every runner's hope is to be able to run through an injury, we all need to pay close attention to painful hamstrings. The pain is likely due to a small tear in the muscle or the tendon. Depending on the severity of the injury, there may be built-up scar tissue, which will further shorten the affected muscle fibers. Hamstring injuries tend to be stubborn, slow to heal, and susceptible to recurrence, so prevention is the best strategy. Once an injury has occurred, gentle stretching and strengthening are helpful during the healing phase; however, overdoing it can make the injury worse. The stretch should be only to the point of no pain, erring on the side of caution to be safe.

In addition to being tight, hamstrings often are also weak. A muscle that is overly tight is also weak because it is not able to move through its full range of motion. In addition to improving the flexibility of your hamstrings, you should also include strengthening work. For all of these reasons, adding a sound and effective hamstrings stretch and strength workout to your plan is essential.

RUNNING, YOGA, AND THE HAMSTRINGS

Just about every style of yoga involves forward bending. If done properly, forward bending is an effective way to stretch the hamstrings and the back muscles. If done incorrectly, forward bending can put a strain on the lower back and on the hamstrings. Ironically, those with the tightest hamstrings need to stretch the most, but they also need to exercise the most caution while doing so. Hamstrings need to be stretched carefully, mindfully, and consistently.

Learning to bend forward properly is necessary for a safe yoga practice, and this increased body awareness will transfer into daily tasks. Either due to tight hamstrings and back muscles, or from habit, the tendency is to initiate the forward bend by moving the upper body forward and rounding the back. Pressing forward from this position puts a strain on both the lower back and the hamstrings, especially if picking up a heavy object.

The safe way to move forward is to hinge forward from the hips and pull the navel in so the abdominals can support the lower back; the feet should be firmly grounded, and the front of the thighs should be contracted (figure 9.2). When lifting heavy objects, the legs can be bent, but in a yoga pose the legs should be straight unless there is pain in the lower back, in which case bending the legs is advised. It is important to move the torso as one unit and to keep the natural curves of the spine in place.

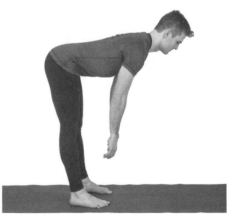

▶ **Figure 9.2** Proper forward bending.

There is a phenomenon in yoga known as overstretching the hamstrings, and sadly, it is a fairly common yoga injury. Picture this scenario: You have tight hamstrings, and after a yoga class, they hurt. You tell yourself that they hurt because they are tight and that with time the pain will go away. You may even try to deepen the hamstring stretches or do more of them. Weeks or months pass, and rather than subsiding, the pain gets worse. At this point, the red flag is raised, and you question whether you are doing the right thing.

When stretching the hamstrings, it is important to stretch the belly of the muscle and avoid tugging at, or aggravating the tendons. The belly is the thickest part of the muscle. The tightness is concentrated in this muscle mass, and these are the muscle fibers that need to be stretched to restore overall length to the hamstrings. However, when the hamstrings are tight, the muscle fibers resist stretching, passing the stretch off to the tendons. A similar effect also results from aggressively stretching the hamstrings or stretching beyond their capacity and ignoring any related pain. Tendons attach muscle to bone and do not have much stretch capacity. Repeating this action will result in overstretching the hamstrings, straining, or even tearing, the tendon. The result is typically a sharp pain at the sitting bones while walking, running, or sitting. This is not an injury to be run through; it needs to be tended to, to restore health to the hamstrings.

Mindfulness and caution are required to safely stretch the hamstrings, particularly during standing forward bends. It is vital to stay tuned to body sensations and to be aware of where along the hamstrings the stretch is occurring. The stretch should be felt in the main body of the hamstrings rather than at either the upper or lower tendons. Any sharpness or discomfort at the sitting bones or the back of the knee is a sign of danger; if this happens, ease the stretch.

An additional safety feature to protect the hamstrings in standing forward bends is to contract the quadriceps, particularly the inner quads (see chapter 10). As antagonist muscles to the hamstrings, contracted quads help the hamstrings stretch safely while preventing hyperextension of the knee joint. Furthermore, this strengthens the inner quadriceps, a muscle typically weak in runners and crucial for healthy knee joints.

Tight hamstrings are also weak hamstrings. Strong and healthy muscles contract when they are worked, release and relax when they are at rest, and lengthen through a reasonable range so as not to create misalignment. Perpetually tight hamstrings are weak, making them more prone to injury and also susceptible to muscle imbalances with the hips and the quads.

Stretching alone is not enough. In yoga you also seek to consciously contract the hamstrings, which supports and creates ease and stability in various poses. Hamstrings that are balanced in strength and flexibility keep the spine in proper alignment, relieve lower-back pain, and help stabilize the hips. Taking care of your hamstrings will pay big dividends in reducing your risk of injury while maintaining a long, fluid, and efficient stride, and you will no longer be sidelined at races with nasty hamstring spasms.

YOGA POSES FOR THE HAMSTRINGS

The poses in this section are for stretching and strengthening the hamstrings.

Hamstrings Eccentric Stretch

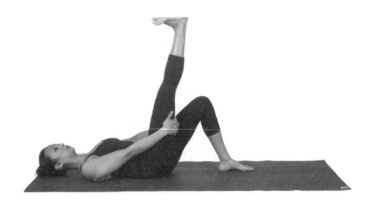

Description

1. Lie supine with the legs bent.
2. Extend, lift, and straighten the right leg and clasp the hands around the thigh or calf.
3. Strongly pull the leg toward you and at the same time, strongly press it away from you into the hands.
4. The more resistance you create, the deeper the stretch will be.

Benefits

- Stretches the hamstrings while they maintain tension, so they are less apt to overstretch
- Is a good stretch in cases of acute hamstring injury or for those prone to over-stretching

Hamstrings Curl

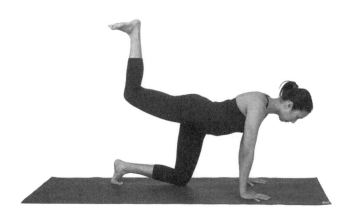

Description

1. Start on hands and knees as in the cat–dog stretch (chapter 7), in a neutral spine position.
2. Lift the left leg, bending it to 90 degrees, with the ankle over the knee, the thigh in line with the hip, and the foot flexed. Do not let the weight shift to the left.
3. Consciously contract the hamstrings and slowly move the leg upward about 6 to 10 inches (15 to 25 cm). As you press the thigh upward, imagine that you are pressing into resistance. Release the thigh to hip height and repeat the pulsing action. Keep the hips square and do not let the weight shift.
4. Do not move with momentum; rather use a slow controlled movement.
5. Repeat on the other side.

Variation

1. This pose can also be done lying prone with a bent or straight leg (as in locust pose in chapter 7).

Benefits

- Strengthens the hamstrings
- Strengthens the glutes

Standing Forward Bend

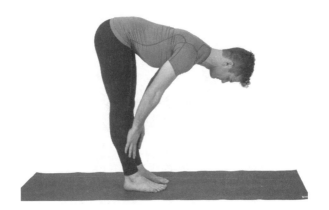

Description

1. From equal standing (chapter 6), step the feet hip-distance apart with the outer edges of the feet parallel, the hands on the hips, and the elbows in to open the chest.

2. Hinging from the hip joints, fold forward, lengthening the front of the torso and keeping the spine neutral. Bend only to the point at which you feel a mild to moderate hamstrings stretch and the back is not rounded.

3. Lengthen the spine by extending the sides of the torso. Let the hands slide down the thighs or shins; do not round the back.

4. Keep the head in line with the shoulders and the back of the neck long and relaxed.

5. Press the feet firmly into the floor, contract the quadriceps, and lift the sitting bones toward the ceiling. Note that if there is lower-back pain, bend the legs slightly.

6. To come up, lengthen the breastbone forward, pull in the navel, press the sitting bones down, and come to an upright position.

Variation

1. Place a belt under the bases of toes. As you fold forward, wrap the hands around the belt and pull up.

Benefits

- Stretches the hamstrings, calves, and hips.
- Strengthens the quadriceps and knees.
- Lengthens the spinal and back muscles.

Triangle

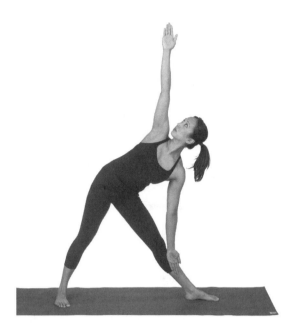

Description

1. From equal standing (chapter 6), step the feet about 4 feet (1.2 m) apart. Raise and straighten the arms to shoulder height, with the shoulder blades down the back and the palms down.

2. Turn the right toes out to 90 degrees and the left foot in slightly. Align the feet so that the center of the front heel is in line with the center of the back arch.

3. Externally rotate the right thigh so that the center of the right kneecap is in line with the center of the right ankle. Contract the quadriceps.

4. Slide the hips to the left as you lengthen the right side of the torso over the right leg.

5. Rotate the right ribs forward to open the chest, and try to keep the two sides of the body equally long. Lengthen the tailbone toward the back heel and pull in the navel.

6. Rest the right hand on the shin without putting any weight on it. Stretch the left arm toward the ceiling. Keep the head in a neutral position, or turn it to softly gaze at the left hand.

7. To come up, press into the feet and lift to upright from the abdomen. Pivot the feet and repeat on the other side.

Benefits

- Stretches the hamstrings, adductors, and calves
- Strengthens the thighs, knees, and ankles
- Stretches the shoulders, chest, and spine

Straight-Leg Lunge

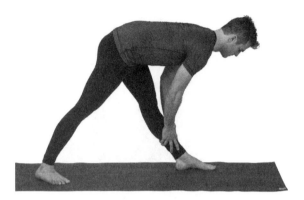

Description

1. Coming into the pose from equal standing (chapter 6), take a step back with the left leg, place the foot at 45 to 65 degrees, and press the heel to the floor.

2. Align the inner front heel with the outer back heel. The length of a stride is about 4 feet (1.2 m), but adjust this so that the back heel remains on the floor.

3. Keep the hips square, back leg straight, and front leg as straight as possible. Contract the quads and align the center of the front kneecap with the center of the ankle.

4. With the hands at the hips, lengthen the spine, slide the breastbone forward, and fold forward, hinging from the hips. Elongate the sides of the torso over the front leg. Let the hands slide down the front leg toward the floor, but do not let the back round or the back heel lift.

5. Keep the head in line with the shoulders.

6. To come up, lift the abdomen, extend the breastbone forward, and return to an upright position.

7. Switch legs and repeat on the other side.

Variation

1. This pose can also be done with the back foot front facing, resting on toe bases with the heel off the ground and pressing toward the floor. Hips are square.

Benefits

- Stretches the hamstrings, calves, and Achilles tendon
- Lengthens the spinal and back muscles
- Strengthens the legs

Revolved Triangle

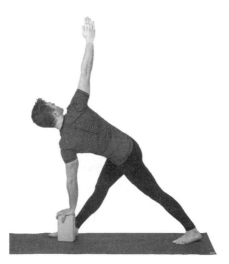

Description

1. Set up as in the straight-leg lunge.
2. It is helpful to have a block for this pose, placing it at the inner front ankle. Move into this pose as you would for straight-leg lunge, but place the left hand on the floor or on the block, and rest the right hand at the lower back.
3. Pressing firmly into the hand, rotate the torso to the right, turning from the base of the spine through the entire length of the spine and keeping the spine long and breastbone extended forward.
4. Keep the hips square and outer hips contracted for stability, the back heel grounded, the legs straight, and the quads firm.
5. Lengthen from the pubic bone to the navel and from the navel to the breastbone, and keep the head aligned with the shoulders. If an adequate degree of rotation is achieved, the right arm can extend to the ceiling to help open the chest. If this is difficult, keep the hand at the lower back.
6. To come up, press the hand into the block, extend the breastbone forward, pull in the navel, and return to standing.
7. Switch legs and repeat on the other side.

Benefits

- Stretches the hamstrings, calves, and Achilles tendon
- Stretches the iliotibial band (IT band)
- Stretches the spinal and back muscles
- Mobilizes and energizes the spine
- Strengthens the legs
- Improves balance
- Opens the chest

Standing Wide-Leg Forward Bend

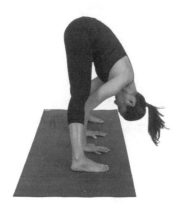

Description

1. From equal standing (chapter 6), step the feet about 5 feet (1.5 m) apart. Turn the toes in so the outer edges of the feet are parallel. Lift the inner ankles and press the big toe joints firmly into the floor to activate the arches of the feet. Contract the quadriceps and adductors (inner thighs), creating a lifting sensation from the inner knees to the inner groins.

2. Rest the hands on the hips, lift the chest, and hinge forward from the hips. As the torso approaches parallel to the floor, press the fingertips or palms into the floor directly below the shoulders and straighten the arms. Lengthen the sides of the torso keeping the spine in a neutral position (not rounded).

3. Deepen the forward fold and walk the hands between the feet only if you are able to move forward from the hips without rounding the back. Bend the elbows and lower the torso and head into a deeper forward bend.

4. Press the shoulders away from the ears.

5. To come up, bring the hands back to the floor below the shoulders, lift and lengthen the spine, and slide the breastbone forward. Bring the hands to the hips, pull in the navel, press the sitting bones down, and lift the torso to an upright position.

6. Return to equal standing.

Benefits

- Stretches the hamstrings and adductors
- Stretches the spine
- Strengthens the arches of the feet
- Strengthens the quads and adductors

Gate

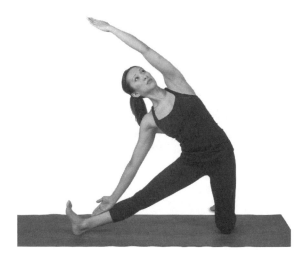

Description

1. Kneel on the floor, with extra padding under the knee if required.
2. Extend the right leg to the right, aligning the foot with the right hip and pressing the heel to the floor, foot flexed. Point the kneecap toward the ceiling, with the inner thigh rotating upward. Keep the extended leg straight, but be sure to contract the quadriceps to avoid hyperextension of the knee joint.
3. Keep the hips square and the left knee directly below the left hip.
4. Raise the arms to shoulder height with palms down. Extend the torso to the right, letting the right hand slide along the leg. Keep the right buttock tucked under.
5. Extend the left arm overhead and reach through the fingertips. Press the shoulder blades down the back.
6. Open the chest toward the ceiling.
7. To come up, pull in the navel and reach through the top arm to draw the torso upright.
8. Place hands on the floor, bring the right leg back to starting position and repeat on the other side.

Benefits

- Stretches the sides of the torso and the spine
- Stretches the obliques
- Stretches the hamstrings, especially the lower muscle fibers
- Strengthens the quadriceps

Seated Forward Bend

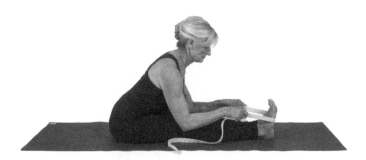

Description

1. Start in staff pose (chapter 7). If the hips tilt back, sit on a folded blanket or block. Have a strap by your side.

2. Straighten the legs, roll the thighs inward, and flex the feet.

3. Lengthen the torso by lifting from the base of the spine. Roll the upper arm bones back as you slide the shoulder blades down the back, and bend forward from the hips, letting the hands move toward the feet. If the hands cannot get to the feet without rounding the back, place a strap at the base of the toes. As you pull the strap, lengthen the breastbone forward. If there is lower-back pain, bend the legs slightly.

4. Keep the sitting bones firmly grounded, and draw the navel in.

5. Do not forcefully pull into the forward bend. Rather, lengthen the front and sides of the torso, keeping the head in line with the shoulders.

6. To come up, reach forward through the breastbone and lift the torso.

Benefits

- Stretches the hamstrings and calves
- Stretches the back muscles
- Stretches the spine—the lower back in particular

Seated Wide-Leg Forward Bend

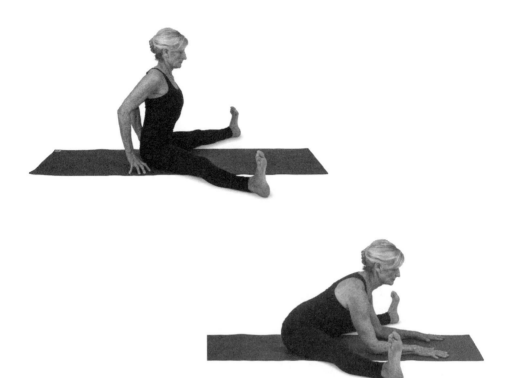

Description

1. From staff pose (chapter 7), open the legs to a wide stance, a little less than your maximum. If the hips tilt back, sit on a folded blanket or block.
2. Straighten the legs, rotate the upper thighs outward, and press them firmly to the floor with the kneecaps pointing toward the ceiling.
3. Flex the feet and reach out through the heels.
4. Fold forward by moving from the hips, and extend the arms forward to lengthen the sides of the body. As the arms extend forward, pull the shoulder blades down the back.
5. To come up, reach the breastbone forward and lift up with a long torso, bring the legs together, and return to staff pose.

Benefits

- Stretches the hamstrings and adductors
- Stretches the spine and back muscles
- Stretches the inner thighs and groins

Supine Hamstrings Stretch

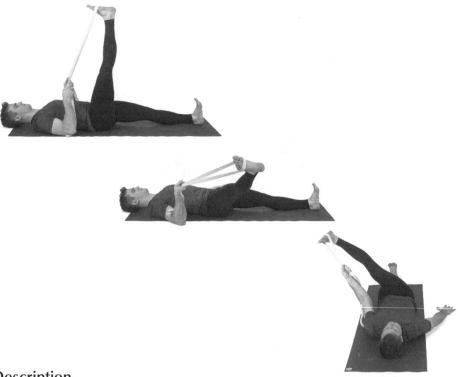

Description

1. **Part 1:** Lie supine with the feet together, legs fully extended, and arms by the sides. Bend the right knee toward the chest and wrap a strap around the toe bases of the right foot. Raise the leg and straighten it so there is no bend in the knee.

2. Flex the foot and press the sitting bone forward to lengthen the lower back.

3. Press the left hand firmly on the left thigh to press it into the floor and rotate it inwardly.

4. Relax the shoulders. Hold.

5. **Part 2:** Next, take the belt in the right hand and open the right leg to the right, aiming the foot toward the right shoulder. Press out through the heel and keep the leg straight. Keep the left hip grounded and leg strongly engaged. Hold.

6. **Part 3:** Finally, take the belt in the left hand and move the right leg to the left, keeping the right hip on the floor. Reach out through the heel, and extend the right hip crease forward to lengthen the waist. Hold.

7. Return the leg to center and release to the floor.

8. Repeat on the other side.

Benefits

- Stretches the hamstrings, hips, inner thighs, inner groins, and calves
- Stretches the iliotibial band (final movement only)

Chapter 10

Hips: Unleash the Power

When using the term *hips,* it is used as a generic term referring to the hip region, also known as the pelvis or pelvic girdle. The hip joint, where the femur bone attaches to the hip bone, is the key joint in this region. Examining the human skeleton, we can clearly see that the hips have an important role in our body structure. They are the interface between the upper and lower body, pivotal in creating movement, and the home of our center of gravity. Tightness in the hips is a common malady among the general population, and perhaps more so for runners. This is not surprising, given that when we sit, the pelvis is weight bearing and the hip joint is locked, leaving this part of the body susceptible to becoming overly tight, stagnant, and a source of pain, discomfort, and injury.

In addition to causing overall pain and discomfort in the hip region, tight hips and muscular imbalances can affect the spine, the knees, and even the shoulders. Moreover, tight hips affect a runner's stride. In addition to increasing mobility in the hips, runners also need to strengthen the muscles that stabilize the hips. Along with a strong core, strong and stable hips reduce the impact of body weight on the lower limbs. This chapter describes the structure of the hip region and the ill effects tightness has on it, and outlines poses to increase mobility and strengthen this vital part of the body.

STRUCTURE OF THE HIP

The hips are heavily packed with muscles and tendons that create the stability needed for weight bearing while also allowing for necessary movement. The dominant action of sitting keeps the hip joint locked in one position, and although walking and running require some degree of movement, that movement is within the same plane. Over time, the range of motion in the hip joint is lost, and the simple action of sitting cross-legged on the floor becomes a daunting task.

The hip joint, being of ball-and-socket construction, has a tremendous range of motion in several planes. Consider the yogi who can wrap both legs behind his head (known as the yogi's sleep pose) or the dancer who can fully extend her leg parallel to her upper body. These demonstrate the possible, though extreme, ranges of motion of the hip joint. Somewhere between the extreme mobility and overly stiff ranges lies a moderate range of motion to strive for. This results in a healthy hip joint that can move through a reasonable range of motion, leaving you able to sit cross-legged on the floor with relative ease.

Many hours a day spent sitting, standing, or walking contributes to a loss of range of motion in the hip joint. The femur bone loses its ability to externally rotate, which results in what we generally refer to as tight hips. During running, many muscles related to the hip joint, especially the external rotators, are overused, shorten, and further contribute to tightening the hip joint. Tight hip flexors and weak glutes add further dysfunction to the hip region.

Hip pain is common among runners and can range from mild, occasional discomfort to deep and chronic pain that can affect the ability to walk, run, or sit. In addition to the annoying aches and pains related to muscle tightness or strain, more severe problems such as stress fractures, arthritis, and nerve compression can arise. Tightness and weakness in the hips contributes to musculoskeletal imbalances, which can affect posture as well as cause lower-back pain, knee problems, and other lower-extremity injuries.

Tightness and weakness in the hips can wreak havoc for runners, leading to any number of injuries. Tight hips limit hip extension and the forward movement of the legs, resulting in a shortened stride. A long and fluid stride is replaced with a choppy and uneven movement. Along with adequate core strength, strong and stable hips have the crucial role of stabilizing the body during movement. The more stable the hips are, the more efficient the running stride will be and the lower the impact of body weight will be on the legs.

To move through your daily tasks, you need a healthy and balanced body with an adequate range of motion in the hip joints so you can move from sitting to standing without creaking, walk and run without unnecessary limitation, and be free of pain while doing so. Strong and flexible hips ease everyday movements and improve running biomechanics. Healthy hips require a balance of flexibility and strength—adequate range of motion in all intended planes and sufficient strength for stability.

As earlier described, the pelvis is made up of a number of bones, muscles, tendons, and joints. The hip joint (figure 10.1) is part of this region and is one of the largest joints in the body. Its primary function is to support the weight of the body while standing, walking, or running. The ball-and-socket structure of the hip joint provides its tremendous range of motion.

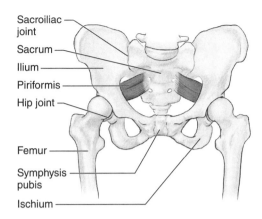

▶ **Figure 10.1**   The hips.

Over 30 muscles attach to the hips in one form or another, and many of these are important in running. Some of these muscle groups have been discussed in previous chapters, including the core, spine, and hamstrings. This chapter examines a smaller group that more directly relates to the pelvis and is especially important for runners, although by no means is this an exhaustive list of muscles.

External Rotators   Reduced range of motion in the hip joints is mostly related to tight external rotators, a group of six muscles also known as the deep six because of their location deep in the pelvis. As implied by their name, their primary function is the external rotation of the hip joint. Keeping the hip joint locked in one position, as in sitting or standing, is a leading cause of tightness, but running shortens these muscles further because of the increased demand for stability from these muscles while running. The increased forward momentum of the legs demands that the rotators contract to hold the pelvis level. With every step that pounds the foot into the ground, these muscles contract to stabilize the body.

Sitting cross-legged on the floor is perhaps the simplest way to use the external rotators. If this is challenging, do it daily to regain this range of motion. If it is comfortable for you, keep doing it so you retain this range. A typical yoga practice offers many opportunities to stretch the muscles in this key group.

Flexors   Flexion is when the upper body and lower body move toward each other, such as when we are sitting, climbing stairs, or bending forward. You are probably in some degree of flexion a majority of the time. You rise and walk around getting ready for the day, perhaps sit as you commute to work, sit at a computer for hours on end, run, and sit to watch television. During all these actions, your hip flexors are contracted. Tight hip flexors will misalign the hips, pulling them into anteversion, or downward, increasing the lower-back arch and causing the abdomen to protrude.

The major hip flexors of the body are the quadriceps (described in further detail in chapter 6) and the iliopsoas (described in further detail in chapter 8). Most runners know they have tight hamstrings or hips, but most are not as familiar with the front of their bodies. Quad stretching can be somewhat awkward and is often painful, which is why many avoid it. Nonetheless, it is a vital muscle group that needs to be balanced in strength and flexibility to restore balance to the body.

Other than lunges, most quad stretching poses require the leg to bend into deep flexion. Caution and safety must be exercised when doing these types of poses. An intense stretch felt in the belly of the quadriceps is safe; however, any pulling or tugging at the knee may be stretching the tendon and should be avoided.

Gluteals The gluteals include the gluteus maximus, gluteus medius, and gluteus minimus, and together they are commonly referred to as the glutes. The gluteus maximus is the largest of the three and the one that gives the desired shape to nicely filled-out our jeans. The gluteus medius is smaller and mostly lies beneath the gluteus maximus. For those who love to run and do little else, the glutes are weak, giving rise to what's called the dead butt syndrome. The glutes are vital for strength and stability in the pelvis. Furthermore, when they are weak, the body compensates by overworking other muscles, leading to other muscular imbalances.

In recent years, the gluteus medius has received more attention, and its role in running has become better understood. For anyone prone to repeated injury in the legs, including the knees, ankle, shins, or feet, it is worth exploring the benefits of strengthening the gluteus medius. Strong gluteus medius muscles are vital to maintaining good running form, eliminating nagging hip pain, and reducing the risk of injury. Like any muscle, the gluteus medius needs to have a balance of strength and flexibility. Yoga offers ample opportunities to strengthen and stretch this muscle through a range of poses. However, if this muscle is weak, it will not kick in and other muscles will compensate. Unlike its showy cousin the gluteus maximus, the gluteus medius requires some concentrated effort to locate. For most, it needs to be awoken and consciously contracted until it learns to fire automatically. It is best to learn to contract these muscles by isolating them, becoming familiar with the feeling during active contraction, and then mindfully contracting them in yoga poses.

FINDING THE GLUTEUS MEDIUS

The following instructions will teach you how to isolate and contract the gluteus medius so you can mindfully do so in many of the standing poses, especially lunges, and in balancing poses. In addition to helping your running, using these muscles will stabilize your yoga poses so that you can hold them for a period of time with little effort.

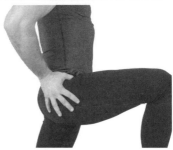

1. From the knees, step the right foot forward so the leg is bent at 90 degrees, and the knee is over the ankle.

2. Slide the thumb of the right hand in the hip crease with the palm resting flat at the outer hip joint. You will feel the gluteus medius beneath the palm.

3. Consciously contract beneath your palm. If you are able to do so, you will feel the outer hip become firmer and contract inward slightly. This is often described as a feeling of compactness at the hip joint.

4. If you are able to feel the contraction, hold for several seconds and repeat a few times. If you are unable to feel the contraction, keep doing so; with focused concentration, eventually the muscle will respond.

5. Repeat on the other side. It is not uncommon for one side to be different from the other.

This directs your mind to the gluteus medius so you can consciously contract it. Over time, you will be able to contract it with less difficulty in poses when needed.

• •

Tensor Fasciae Latae (TFL)   The tensor fasciae latae (TFL) is a short muscle and starts at the top front outer hip bone (known as the iliac crest). Its function is abduction, internal rotation, and hip flexion. The TFL connects to a long band of tissue called the iliotibial band (IT band), which runs along the side of the leg and attaches below the knee. A tight TFL contributes to iliotibial band syndrome (ITB), a very common running injury. A tight TFL can also be the cause of hip and knee pain. Tight hip flexors and weak gluteal muscles require the TFL to work overtime. Thus, the TFL is a small but important muscle to pay attention to.

Adductors   The adductors are a group of muscles located at the inner thighs, and as the name suggests, their primary function is to adduct (i.e., bring the legs together). They are powerful muscles that are key in stabilizing the pelvis in movement. In many runners, the adductors are tight and weak, contributing to muscular imbalance. Adductors are used in actions such as horseback riding, which for many of us are uncommon, leaving this muscle group prone to being weak. Yet to be balanced in leg strength and stable in the hips and knees, these muscles need to be stretched and strengthened.

Luckily, yoga offers ample opportunities to do both. Many yoga poses require the contraction of the adductors to support the legs through various moves. However, because this muscle group tends to be weak, contracting these muscles requires mindful effort and attention to alignment detail. The result is balanced leg strength, which for runners translates into fewer injuries and stronger running.

RUNNING, YOGA, AND THE HIPS

Yoga is a balm for tight hips and a great way to combat the effects of both sitting and running. Most yoga poses have some effect on the hips. For example, some poses require the hips to remain in neutral, which may sound simple but can be very challenging. This challenge provides a dynamic blend of strengthening and stretching. In other poses we try to move the hips in a particular direction, or stabilize the hips and move the femur bones, which stretches out tight spots. A balanced yoga practice stretches the overused and tightened muscles, giving the hip joint the freedom it needs to move unencumbered. With the right attention to detail, yoga also strengthens the muscles that support the hip joint, creating the pelvic balance and stability required for efficient and fluid weight transfer.

Hip poses can be very challenging for athletic bodies, yet perseverance pays off because the positive effects of a good hip-opening session are felt immediately. Runners often comment that their running stride feels more fluid and their bodies feel lighter after a hip-centered yoga class.

Yet care and attention needs to be paid to hip work in yoga. When the hip joint is tight and limited in its range of motion, the movement will tend to transfer to the knee joint. Recall that the knee joint is a simple joint that serves only as a hinge. Yoga poses that require external rotation must focus on moving the femur bone at the hip joint while letting the knee rest where it lands. For example, when sitting in a simple cross-legged position, the knees will be far away from the floor or even pointed to the ceiling if the hips are tight. The knees of those with greater hip mobility are closer to the floor. Although you may be tempted to do so, never press down on the knees! The knees will come to rest where the range of motion of the hip joint permits. Pushing beyond the point at which hip mobility permits will torque the knee beyond its available range. If done repeatedly, the knee joint will start

Emma's Story

After running a few years and having completed a marathon and triathlon, and while training for my next marathon, my left hip was really starting to bother me. It was diagnosed as bursitis. Shortly after this I learned about *Yoga for Runners*, and that is what got me into yoga. Years later, with 10 marathons completed, yoga has become such an integral part of my life that it's hard to remember "pre-yoga." My overall strength and flexibility have increased tremendously, and I have not had a running injury since. I look forward to my yoga practices as much as I do my running. I am convinced that yoga has helped me keep the injuries at bay!

to hurt, usually at the inner knee. Over time, and with a consistent yoga practice, the mobility of the hip joint will improve and the knees will release closer to the floor. You cannot rush this process! It is important to move safely and mindfully through yoga poses so the hips receive the desired effect without putting the knees at risk.

YOGA POSES FOR THE HIPS

The poses in this section are for stretching and strengthening the hips. Because so many muscles affect the hip joint, it is important to include a variety of hip poses into a yoga practice. Therefore, some of the exercises are not technically yoga poses, but actions that complement the yoga poses.

Quadriceps and Iliotibial Band Rollouts

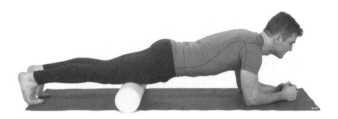

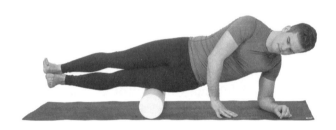

Description

1. Lie prone on a foam roller, placing the roller under the quadriceps.
2. Press the forearms into the floor and roll forward and back, sliding along the roller from the top to the bottom of the thighs. Do not roll over the knees or hip joints.
3. Repeat several times.
4. Roll to one side and continue rolling along the side of the upper thigh for a deep massage effect on the iliotibial band. Repeat several times.
5. Repeat on the other side.
6. For both rollouts:
   - Start with the feet resting on the floor, but eventually bring the feet off the floor with both legs straight.
   - As you roll out the length of the front and sides of the thighs, you will likely encounter one or two spots that are particularly painful. Rather than avoid such a spot, remain here and release your body weight into the roller to allow the tight spot to soften.

Benefits

- Releases tightness in the quadriceps and iliotibial band
- Soothingly self-massages tight muscles
- Increases the flexibility of the muscles that attach to the iliotibial band
- Breaks down the tiny lesions that form between the muscles and the fascia

Kneeling Clam

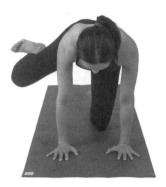

Description

1. Set up as in the cat–dog stretch (chapter 7).
2. Consciously contract the outer left hip (gluteus medius) to keep the hips square.
3. Pull in the navel to stabilize the core.
4. Lift the right knee off the ground a few inches, and keeping the ankle and knee aligned, lift the leg away from the body (abduct).
5. Move only as far as possible without letting the weight shift to the left. Return the right knee so it almost touches the left one and repeat this lifting action.
6. If the hips start to sway, take a rest with both knees on the floor; then try again.
7. Move slowly, mindfully, and with control rather than momentum.
8. Return the knee to the floor and repeat on the other side.

Benefits

- Strengthens the gluteus medius and gluteus maximus
- Strengthens the core

Tabletop With Leg Extended

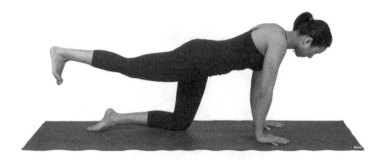

Description

1. Set up as in kneeling clam. Extend the right leg straight, in line with the hip and spine. Keep the extended leg very straight and firm with the foot flexed.
2. Contract the outer left hip (gluteus medius) to keep the hips square.
3. Pull in the navel to stabilize the core.
4. Move the extended leg up and down about 6 inches (15 cm) in a pulsing action, contracting the gluteus maximus so it is firmest at the top of the pulse.
5. Repeat on the other side.

Variations

1. Once you have completed the pulsing action, keep the leg straight, in line with the hip, and the hips square.
2. Extend the opposite arm, pulling the arm bone into the socket. Look toward the hand.
3. Repeat on the other side.

Benefits

- Strengthens the gluteus medius and gluteus maximus
- Strengthens the core

Downward Dog (Leg Extended Variation)

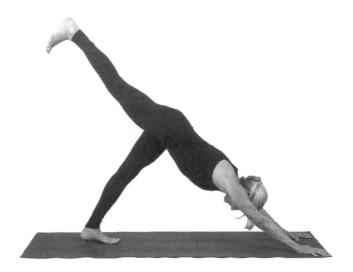

Description

1. Start in downward dog (see chapter 7). Lift and extend the right leg, keeping it straight and in line with the hips.
2. Contract the outer left hip (gluteus medius) to keep the hips square.
3. Pull in the navel and press the shoulder blades into the body to stabilize the core.
4. Lift the leg as high as possible without letting the hips tilt. Slowly lower the foot to the floor.
5. Repeat on the other side.

Benefits

- Strengthens the gluteus medius
- Stretches the piriformis
- Stretches the spine
- Strengthens the upper body

Extended Side Stretch

Description

1. From equal standing (chapter 6), step feet about 5 feet (1.5 m) apart. Raise the arms parallel to the floor and actively extend them to the sides, with shoulder blades down the back and palms down.

2. Turn the left toes out to 90 degrees and the right foot in slightly. Align the feet so that the center of the front heel is in line with the center of the back arch.

3. Anchor the outer edge of the right foot to the floor by lifting the inner arch of the foot and strongly contracting the inner thigh (adductors) from above the knee to the inner groin. Hold this action as you bend the left leg until the left knee is over the left ankle and the shin is perpendicular to the floor. Try to bring the left thigh parallel to the floor, but do not let the knee move inward.

4. Rest the left elbow on the right knee, and roll the left ribs forward and the right ribs to the ceiling to open the chest.

5. Without letting the right sitting bone protrude, lower the hand to the floor, continuing to open the chest. If you are unable to hold the alignment of the hips, keep the elbow at the knee.

6. Press the shoulder blades against the upper back.

7. Extend the right arm overhead, palm facing down. Try to keep upper arm in line with the ear.

8. Pressing the outer foot to the floor, stretch from the right heel through to the right fingertips, lengthening the entire right side of the body.

9. Actively wrap the left sitting bone under by engaging the glutes while keeping the knee fixed over the ankle.

10. To come up, push both feet strongly into the floor and reach the right arm toward the ceiling.

11. Pivot the feet and repeat on the other side.

Benefits

- Stretches the external rotators
- Strengthens the adductors (inner thighs)
- Strengthens and stretches the legs, knees, and ankles
- Stretches the groins, spine, waist, and shoulders
- Strengthens the gluteus medius and gluteus maximus

Bound Side Stretch

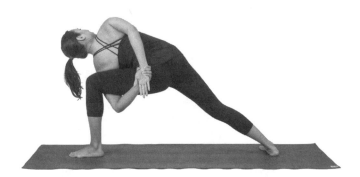

Description

1. Set up as for the extended side stretch.
2. Place the left hand on the floor by the inner ankle, firmly squeeze the shoulder and the inner knee. Inwardly rotate the left upper arm and wrap it under the left thigh. Externally rotate the right arm and wrap it around the lower back, clasping both hands behind the left thigh.
3. Actively contract the inner right thigh, keeping the outer edge of the foot grounded and the inner ankle lifted.
4. Continue to open the chest to the ceiling.
5. To come up, unclasp the hands, press into the feet, and return to upright.
6. Pivot the feet and repeat on the other side.

Benefits

- Stretches the external rotators
- Strengthens the adductors (inner thighs)
- Strengthens and stretches the legs, knees, and ankles
- Stretches the groins, spine, waist, and shoulders
- Strengthens the gluteus medius and gluteus maximus

Warrior II

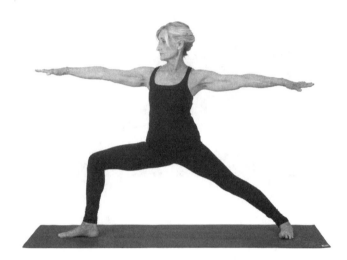

Description

1. Set up as for the extended side stretch.
2. Place the hands on the hip bones and, without letting the hips tilt to the right, bend the right leg so the knee is over the ankle and the shin is perpendicular to the floor. Aim to bring the right thigh parallel to the floor while keeping the knee over the ankle.
3. Keeping the outer left foot grounded, contract the inner left thigh (adductors) from above the knee to the inner groin.
4. Raise the arms to shoulder height, contracting the triceps and pulling the shoulder blades down the back and into the upper rib cage.
5. Don't lean the torso over the front thigh, keep the sides of the torso equally long and the shoulders over the pelvis.
6. Press the sitting bones down and pull the abdomen in. Fix your gaze over the right hand.
7. To come up, press into the feet, straighten the front leg, and pivot the feet.
8. Repeat on the other side.

Benefits

- Stretches the hips
- Strengthens and stretches the inner thighs (adductors)
- Strengthens and stretches the legs and ankles
- Stretches the groins and shoulders
- Strengthens the arms

Standing Egyptian

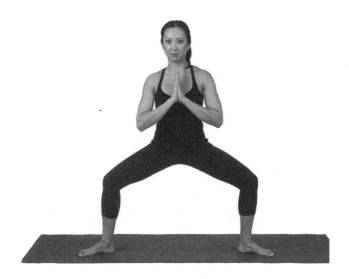

Description

1. From equal standing (chapter 6), step the feet about 5 feet (15 m) apart. Turn the feet out to about 90 degrees.
2. Resting the hands on the thighs, bend the legs while pressing the knees outward and over the ankles.
3. Press the tailbone down and lift the front hip bones. Strongly pull the belly in and lift the breastbone so the upper body is upright.
4. Deepening the bend in the legs will deepen the pose. As the legs bend deeper, the knees will want to turn inward. Keep pressing them outward to align them over the ankles.
5. Arm positions variations include the following:
   - Hands resting on the knees
   - Straight arms raised overhead
   - Hands in prayer
6. To come out of the pose, turn the feet in, straighten the legs, and return to equal standing.

Benefits

- Stretches the external rotators
- Stretches the inner thighs
- Improves balance
- Strengthens the core

Warrior III

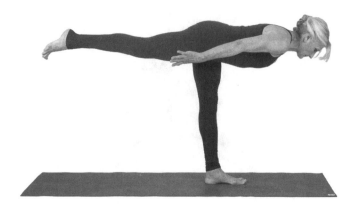

Description

1. Stand at the front of the mat with the hands resting on blocks beneath the shoulders.
2. Stabilize the left leg by grounding the toe bases and heel, contract the quads, lifting from the inner quadriceps to inner groin and contracting the outer left hip (gluteus medius). Pull the navel in.
3. Lift and extend the right leg, keeping it straight and in line with the spine. Do not let the weight shift to the left; keep the hips level.
4. Draw the belly and front ribs in to engage the core, and lift the arms, either by your side, outward in line with the shoulders, or forward with the arms parallel. Hold.
5. Release the extended leg to the floor and bring the feet together.
6. Repeat on the other side.

Benefits

- Strengthens gluteus maximus and gluteus medius
- Stretches the piriformis
- Stretches the hamstrings
- Lengthens the spine
- Strengthens the legs
- Strengthens the core
- Improves balance

Knee to Ankle Balance

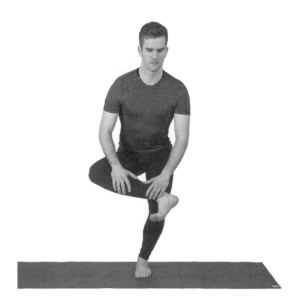

Description

1. From equal standing (chapter 6), bend the right leg and place the outer right ankle above the left knee. Flex the foot.
2. Relax the muscles of the right hip, including the glutes, bend the left leg, and place the hands on the waist, the shins, or the floor.
3. The movement is less of a forward bend and more of a squat.
4. Repeat on the other side.

Benefits

- Stretches the external rotators
- Stretches and strengthens the glutes
- Improves balance and concentration

Tree

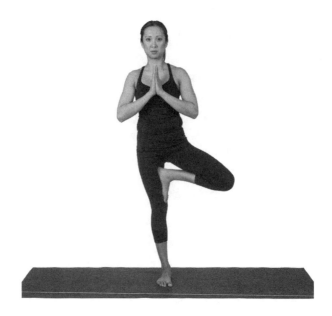

Description

1. Start in equal standing (chapter 6). Bend the right leg and roll the thigh outward.
2. Lift and place the left foot along the inner right thigh, above the knee or below the knee, but not at the knee. If above the knee, press the left foot firmly into the right thigh.
3. Roll the left thigh outward while keeping the hips square and facing front.
4. Turn the left knee to front facing, and release.
5. Repeat on the other side.

Benefits

- Stretches the external rotators
- Stretches and strengthens the inner thighs (adductors)
- Strengthens the legs
- Improves balance and concentration
- Strengthens the ankles

Pigeon

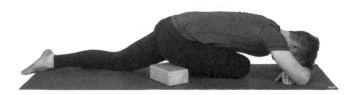

Description

1. From downward dog (chapter 7), slide the right knee to the right hand, and move the right foot and shin upward. Keep the right knee in line with the right hip.
2. Extend the left leg straight back along the floor, and let the right hip rest on the floor, a block, or a folded blanket.
3. Lengthen the upper body and release to the floor, resting the head on folded arms.
4. Relax the shoulders, neck, and head.
5. To come out of the pose, press the hands into the floor, pull navel in to lift the hips, and slide the front leg back to downward dog.
6. Repeat on the other side.

Benefits

- Stretches the external rotators, especially the piriformis
- Stretches the glutes

Double Pigeon

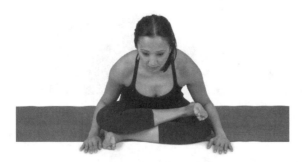

Description

1. Sit in staff pose (chapter 7), bend the right leg, and place the right outer ankle above the left knee. Flex the foot and release the thigh toward the floor.

2. Lean back, bend the left leg, flex the foot, and move the left shin so it is aligned under the right one. Both feet should be flexed.

3. Sit upright with both sitting bones evenly grounded, or move into a forward bend to deepen the stretch.

4. For safety, if the bottom knee is off the ground, the bottom leg can be kept straight, or place a folded blanket underneath for support. Do not let the bottom leg remain suspended without support. If the top knee is higher than the waist, wrap the arms around it to support the pose.

5. Continue to actively press the right thigh downward. Do not press down on the knee; rather, let the work come from the hip.

6. Repeat on the other side.

Benefits

- Opens the hips
- Stretches the glutes

Squat

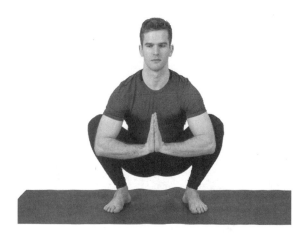

Description

1. Come into this pose from either standing or sitting.
2. From standing, set feet slightly wider than hip distance, toes facing front. Bend the legs, keeping the knees over the ankles, and slowly lower into a squat, ensuring there is no discomfort in the knees.
3. From sitting, set feet as described for standing, shift the weight forward, and lift the hips off the floor.
4. The feet will turn out, but try to keep them as parallel as possible.
5. Let the hips be heavy, and lift the chest to lengthen the spine.

Benefits

- Stretches and decompresses the lower back
- Opens the hips
- Strengthens the shins and ankles
- Stretches the Achilles tendon

Bound Angle

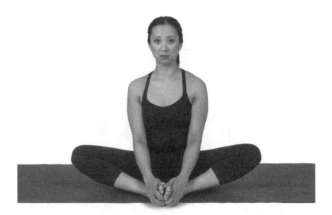

Description

1. Sit in staff pose (chapter 7). Bend the knees and bring the soles of the feet together, heels toward the pelvis.
2. Let the knees fall toward the floor. Press the soles of the feet together and the outside edges of the feet to the floor.
3. If the knees are higher than waist level, sit on one or two blocks.
4. Place the hands behind the back and press them to the floor while pressing the hips forward, dropping the pubic bone to the floor and lifting the sacrum upward.
5. If you can keep the hips upright or forward place the hands on the outer feet.
6. Relax the shoulders and move the shoulder blades down the back. Lengthen the front torso, pull in the abdomen, and lift the chest.
7. Remain upright or move into a forward bend, maintaining a straight spine and open chest.
8. To come out of the pose, bring knees together and straighten the legs.

Benefits

- Opens the hips
- Stretches the external rotators
- Stretches the inner thighs and groins

Internal Rotator Stretch

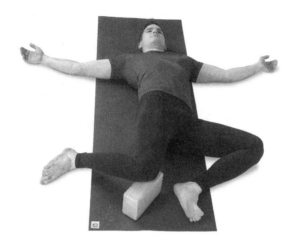

Description

1. Start lying supine with the legs bent to 90 degrees. Slide the right foot to the right about a shin length.

2. Drop the right knee toward the left ankle, letting the thigh rotate inwardly and rest along the inner edge of the foot. The right hip will lift a bit.

3. Ensure the right knee is pointing straight forward and extend the left thigh away from the body.

4. For support place a block or rolled blanket under the right knee, place the outer left ankle on the outer right knee, and pull slightly to the left. If the right knee is far from the floor, or if there is any twinge of discomfort in the knee, skip this step.

5. Repeat on the other side.

Benefits

- Stretches the tensor fasciae latae
- Stretches the gluteus medius

Lunges (Low, Kneeling, and High)

Description

1. To set up for the lunge, from downward dog (chapter 7), step the right foot to the inside of the right hand. Align the right knee over the ankle. Actively press the foot down and contract the hamstrings and the outer right hip (gluteus medius) of the front leg. If you are unable to get the foot to the hand, let the back knee rest on the floor and keep stepping the front foot forward until it reaches the hand; then straighten the back leg. Over time, the foot will move to the hand with greater ease. The front leg is key in stabilizing the lunges. The front knee should remain over the ankle at all times. To come out of the lunge, press hands to the floor beside the front foot, pull the belly in to lift the hips, slide the front leg back, and return to downward dog. Repeat on the other side.

2. For the low lunge *(a)*, keep the hands on the floor by the front foot and straighten the back leg, pressing the heel back. Lift the breastbone, slide the shoulder blades down the back and look up to lengthen the spine.

3. For the kneeling lunge *(b)*, from the setup position, rest the back knee on the floor, placing a folded blanket under the knee if needed. Rest the hands on the front thigh, press down, and draw in the abdomen and lower ribs. Press the tailbone down and lift the front hip bones. Raise the arms overhead, pressing the shoulders down and lifting the chest. To deepen the stretch, move the hips forward while continuing to draw in the abdomen and lower ribs.

4. For the high lunge *(c)*, start from the low lunge and raise the arms overhead. Draw the lower ribs and abdomen in. Press back through the heel and fully straighten the back leg, rolling the inner thigh toward the ceiling. Press the tailbone down and move the front left hip bone forward and upward. Fully straighten the arms to stretch the sides of the torso and spine.

5. To come out of the lunge, place both hands on the floor, raise the hips, step the front foot back, and return to downward dog.

6. Repeat on the other side.

Benefits

- Stretches the hip flexors
- Stretches the calves and Achilles tendon
- Stretches the inner thighs
- Strengthens and stretches the gluteus medius and gluteus maximus
- Strengthens the legs

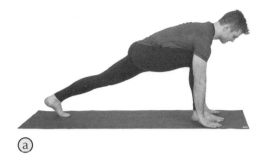

(a)

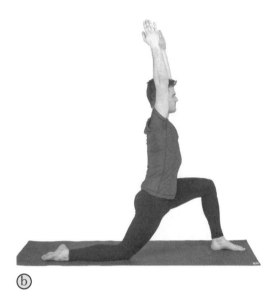

(b)

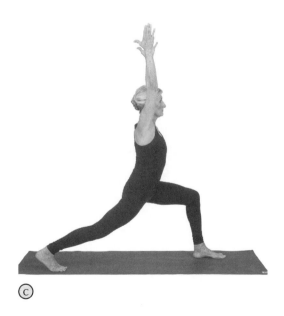

(c)

Lunge Twist

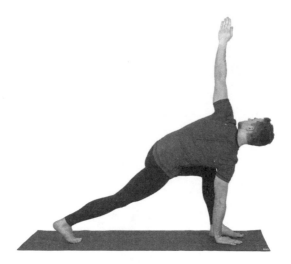

Description

1. From the low lunge position with the left leg forward, place the right hand on the floor beneath the right shoulder and place the left hand at the lower back.

2. Move into a twist by moving from the navel and rolling the right ribs toward the inner left thigh.

3. Press into the right hand, straighten the left arm to the ceiling, and open the chest by lengthening the breastbone forward.

4. To come out, place both hands on the floor, pull the navel in, lift the hips and slide the front leg back to return to downward dog (see chapter 7).

5. Repeat on the other side.

Benefits

- Stretches the hip flexors
- Stretches the calves and Achilles tendon
- Stretches the inner thighs
- Strengthens and stretches the gluteus medius and gluteus maximus
- Strengthens the legs
- Stretches, strengthens, and rejuvenates the spine

Lizard

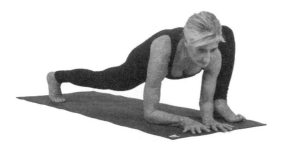

Description

1. From the low lunge position, move the left foot to the left and place the left hand at the inner left foot.

2. Squeeze the left inner thigh toward the body by contracting the inner thigh (adductors).

3. Lengthen the breastbone forward.

4. Bend the elbows gradually and let the forearms rest on the floor or on a yoga block. Do not let the knee sway outward or the right hip drop. Keep the back leg straight.

5. To come out of the pose, press the hands to the floor, lift the hips, and step the front leg back.

6. Repeat on the other side.

Benefits

- Opens the hips
- Stretches and strengthens the inner thighs (adductors)
- Stretches the quadriceps

Twisted Lizard

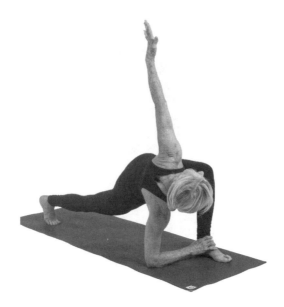

Description

1. Set up in lizard with the elbows on the floor, and let the back knee rest on the floor.
2. Press the right forearm to the floor (or yoga block), and reach for the left ankle with the right hand. Firmly hold on to the left ankle and rest the left hand at the lower back.
3. Create a twisting action by rotating the navel and right ribs toward the left thigh.
4. Raise the left arm and deepen the twist to spiral the chest toward the ceiling.
5. Straighten the back leg, rolling the inner thigh toward the ceiling.
6. To come out of the pose, place both hands on the floor by the front foot, lift hips, and slide the front leg back.
7. Repeat on the other side.

Benefits

- Opens the hips
- Stretches the quads
- Stretches the inner thighs and groins
- Stretches, strengthens, and rejuvenates the spine

Half Frog

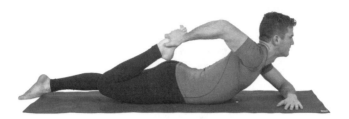

Description

1. Lie prone with the legs straight and press the front hip bones to the floor.
2. Bend the right leg and take the right hand to the top of the foot. Gently press the sole of the foot toward the buttock, keeping hip bone grounded. Ensure there is no excessive tugging or pain at the knee.
3. Place the left arm in front of the body, press the forearm to the floor, pull the navel in, and lift the chest. Press the shoulder blades down.
4. To deepen the stretch, press the femur down and try to lift the thigh from the floor, keeping the front hip bone grounded.

Benefits

- Stretches the quads and hip flexors
- Strengthens the back muscles

Kneeling Quadriceps Stretch

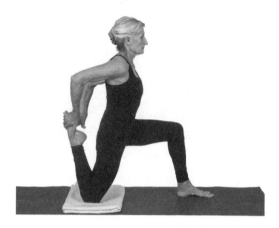

Description

1. Kneeling with a folded blanket under the right knee, step the left leg forward to create a 90 degree angle.

2. Press the hips forward so that the right knee is behind the hips. Place the left hand on the right thigh for balance.

3. Lift the right foot off the floor toward the buttock. Reach back with the right hand and hold onto the top of the foot. Gently draw the right foot toward the buttock while keeping the hips facing forward. Ensure that there is no pain in either knee. The stretch should be felt in the quadriceps.

4. Pull the belly and lower ribs in, and lift the upper body to an upright position. As you deepen the pose, be sure the stretch remains in the quadriceps and front groin with no pain in the knee.

5. To come out of the pose, gently release the back leg, place the hands on the floor, and slide the front leg back so both knees are on the floor.

6. Repeat on the other side.

Variations

1. Hold on to the back foot with both hands, roll the upper arm bones back, and lift the breastbone to open the chest.

2. Hold the right foot with the left hand and straighten the right arm upward, pulling belly and front ribs in.

3. From previous position, twist to the left and rest the outer right hand at the outer left knee. Strongly squeezing the hand and knee together, lift the torso away from the left thigh, keep the upper body upright and continue to deepen the twist.

Benefits

- Stretches the quads
- Stretches the iliopsoas
- Opens the chest

Chapter 11

Quietude and Relaxation: Restore and Recover

Runners are known to be go-getters, doers, and achievers, and they reap many rewards as a result of these characteristics. Maxims such as "Idle hands are the devil's tools" and "Idleness is the root of mischief," which date back to the 14th century, continue to be integrated into today's societal norms. Many of us are on the go from the moment we awaken until we plop into bed at the end of the day. Some of us are physically and mentally exhausted and yet unable to sleep.

Running, with its multitude of health benefits, also provides opportunities to experience the triumphs of going farther and faster. What runner is not interested in improving a past race time, or not constantly moving the yardstick to greater achievements? Most runners also have busy, fulfilling lives in addition to running and often need to plan to squeeze a run in—in the early morning before work, during lunch, or after taking the kids to school. Taking time to rest is simply not on the agenda for many runners. They equate resting to sleeping, and rest only when under the weather.

The preceding chapters discussed the benefits of yoga to various parts of the body. To this point we have focused on strength, flexibility, and a physically active yoga practice. Such a practice has many physical benefits and is essential to keeping the body in balance. However, at times a quieter and more internally calming yoga practice better serves the body and mind. This chapter explores a type of yoga practice known as restorative yoga.

WHAT IS RESTORATIVE YOGA?

Restorative yoga concentrates on resting the body and the mind. The body is arranged in variations of yoga poses and supported with props, allowing the joints to be supported and the muscles to soften and release entirely. This helps the body enter a state of physical relaxation, a deep letting go. At the same time, the mind can shut down from its usual state of pondering, thinking, and musing. You literally enter a state of being rather than doing, which has a tremendously powerful effect on both the body and the mind. An actual rejuvenation occurs within the body.

It is important to note that rest is not the same as sleep. Rest creates an internal environment in which the body can heal and revitalize. If you are accustomed to being active and on the go, you may be drawn to a more physical yoga practice in which you will quickly experience the physical effects. After all, it is easy to feel the hamstrings stretch and understand the benefits. On the other hand, you may well find the thought of being idle and spending an extended period of time in one pose less alluring, if not downright boring. However, I encourage you to give restorative yoga a try without judgment to feel the internal effects for yourself. Students typically express a feeling of inner calm, have reduced stress, forget their problems for a while, and are able to sleep better. Given the high degree of stress experienced in today's world, adding a restorative yoga component to your fitness regimen is a must for optimal health and wellness.

As detailed in chapter 3, yoga's deep breathing stimulates the central nervous system and helps to bring the sympathetic and parasympathetic systems into balance. Restorative yoga poses stimulate the parasympathetic nervous system on a deeper level. This helps to lower heart rate and blood pressure and stimulates the immune system. It also allows the body's own internal healing process to kick in.

As you know, running is very good for you, but as a high-impact exercise, it is hard on the body. The impact of running and the related constant contraction of muscles create micro-tears, which are what cause the leg pain and stiffness after a hard run. These tears are healed by the nutrients supplied by the blood flowing to the muscles. A physical yoga practice enhances this recovery by stimulating the muscles and increasing blood supply. Restorative yoga, although less physical than other forms of yoga, stimulates a more profound level of healing throughout the entire body. It is of tremendous value to runners, aiding recovery from arduous training runs and races while helping injuries to heal more quickly.

When you take the time for even just a few restorative yoga poses, your mind–body connection is strengthened, and you feel the tremendous power deeply. A calm, soothing energy ensues and renews you so you are better able to meet and cope with life's ongoing challenges.

WHEN TO PRACTICE RESTORATIVE YOGA

Finding an ideal time to practice restorative yoga is less important than simply doing it. Work it into your fitness routine in a way that best suits your schedule and your personal preferences. Try it at various times of the day and see which times your body prefers.

Doing a few restorative poses is a great way to prepare for the day. The revitalizing effect on the body and the ensuing mental clarity will carry you through the day with greater ease. Try it on days that you know are likely to be particularly busy and stressful.

A few restorative poses at the end of the day can help release the stresses of the day. When you are unable to turn off thinking, your jaw is tight, your shoulders are full of tension, or you have a tension headache, a calming yoga practice can bring immediate rewards. Restorative yoga just before bedtime is highly recommended if you suffer from insomnia, have difficulty falling asleep, or wake in the middle of the night. The deep, calming effects and slowing down of the body and mind will prepare you for a good nights' sleep. With better sleep, you will feel more rested and revived and have greater energy the following day.

Because of its healing effects, restorative yoga is extremely helpful when dealing with an acute injury. Runners hate to be injured and want to get back on the road as quickly as possible. Furthermore, being injured and unable to run often creates stress and frustration, which only delays the healing. The powerful therapeutic benefits of restorative yoga create an internal environment conducive to healing and speed recovery from injuries.

Restorative yoga is a good way to recover from a race or a particularly grueling training run. When you feel depleted after a run, you may not feel up to a physical yoga practice and understandably forgo it. In a situation such as this, experiment by taking the time to do a few calming poses and note the effects in your body and mind. You can then do your physical yoga practice the following day.

Restorative yoga need not be done solely on its own; it can be integrated into your physical yoga practice. Simply leave yourself some time at the end of your practice for one or two of your favorite restorative poses. Additionally, you will be practicing deep, diaphragmatic breathing, either abdominal or ujjayi, while in your restorative yoga poses. The breathing further stimulates the parasympathetic nervous system and will deepen the relaxation, rejuvenation, and healing process.

As you can see, there is no prescribed formula—no right or wrong time to practice restorative yoga. These suggestions may be helpful initially, but your own intuition will be the best judge. As your body becomes accustomed to the tremendous effects of restorative yoga, it will become your best and most trustworthy guide.

PROPS

Restorative yoga poses require a number of props. Well-equipped yoga studios typically have blankets, bolsters, pillows, yoga blocks, and yoga chairs, which are necessary for a restorative yoga practice that includes many poses. However, a number of restorative poses can be done with makeshift props you can create in your own home.

When placing your props, don't be afraid to move them around until you find that perfect point of comfort. The difference between comfort and pain may be a slight adjustment of the prop here or there. Remember that the purpose of props is to induce comfort; there should be no tension in your body while in the pose. It may take some adjusting of the props until you find the right fit. Listen to your body.

Following is a description of the props needed for the restorative yoga poses described later in the chapter, including how to create your own makeshift props. The number of folds varies depending on the size of your blankets.

Blankets   You will need two blankets approximately the same size, and each one should be a little larger than a yoga mat. Ideally, to serve as a prop, a blanket should be tightly woven so it retains its shape under your body weight. A thick bath towel can also work. The blanket should be neatly folded with even edges, no bumps, and no creases.

- **Folded blanket:** Fold the blanket in half lengthwise and then in half lengthwise two or three more times until it becomes a long folded strip approximately 1 foot (30 cm) wide (figure 11.1). The folds need to be neat to create an even density in the finished product.
- **Rolled blanket:** Fold the blanket in half lengthwise three times. Start at the long edge and roll the blanket to create a neat, even, and dense roll (figure 11.2).

Bolster   A yoga bolster is a large rectangular pillow with an even firmness and density. To create a home bolster, roll the outer edges of a sleeping pillow inward slightly, and firmly wrap the full length with a blanket. You can bind it in place with one or two straps if needed.

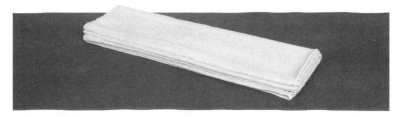

▶ **Figure 11.1**   Blanket fold.

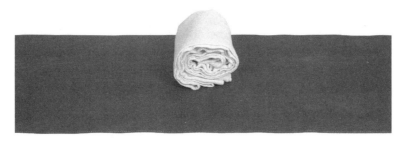

▶ **Figure 11.2**   Blanket roll.

Pillows   One or two pillows are helpful. You can use any you have available, but they should be approximately the same size.

Yoga Blocks   Yoga blocks are typically made of wood or firm cork construction; they are $4 \times 6 \times 9$ inches ($10 \times 15 \times 23$ cm) in size. Foam blocks are also popular, but they provide less stability, especially if they are very lightweight. Of all the props noted, yoga blocks are the most helpful (you will need two of them), because they can also be used during your physical yoga practice. In the absence of yoga blocks, you can use a stack of books fairly even in size and of the size noted.

Eye Pillow   An eye pillow is useful to cover your eyes while in the poses to facilitate release and induce calmness. A folded hand towel works well.

YOGA POSES FOR RESTORATION AND RECOVERY

This section describes some basic restorative poses that provide a balance of forward bending and back bending. They were selected because they are relatively easy to set up and will give you a sense of the experience of calm and tranquility restorative yoga offers. There are many other restorative poses to explore, however. If this form of yoga interests you, find a restorative yoga class in your community or make use of the many written resources available.

General Guidelines for Practice

- Prepare your props and have them at hand as you prepare for the pose.

- Restorative yoga poses must be accompanied by deep breathing to release tension, stimulate the parasympathetic nervous system (involved in healing and nourishing the body), and induce calmness (review chapter 3).

- Falling asleep in the pose is a good sign that your setup is comfortable and that you are relaxed. However, the aim of restorative yoga is to remain awake and allow your body and mind to rest rather than sleep.

- Hold each pose for at least 3 minutes to start. As time permits, you can build up to holding for 10 to 15 minutes.

- Restorative yoga poses are about releasing all physical tension in the muscles and joints. The props should bear your weight, allowing all parts of the body to be tension free. As you release into the pose, do a quick body scan to be sure you are not unknowingly holding tightness. Pay particular attention to your mouth, jaw, neck, shoulders, and abdomen.

Supported Chest Opener

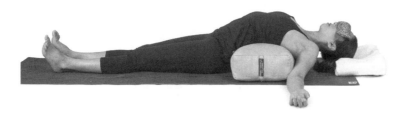

Props

- Bolster
- One pillow
- Eye pillow (optional)

Description

1. Sit at the front of the yoga mat with the legs bent.
2. Place the bolster horizontally so it is positioned at the center of the back. Gently lie over the bolster so the middle back is supported, with the upper arms and shoulders resting over the top of the bolster, releasing toward the floor. The hips should remain on the floor.
3. Let the head fall toward the floor. If the forehead slopes backward, place a small pillow beneath the head. The chin should point toward the chest so that the back of the neck is long and the front of the neck is soft and relaxed.
4. For deeper relaxation, place an eye pillow over the eyes.
5. You may need to adjust the props a few times to find the best positioning for your body.

Variation

1. This pose can also be done with the legs bent, feet wider than hip-distance apart, and knees together; or with the legs crossed; or with the legs straight and feet together.

Supported Bound Angle

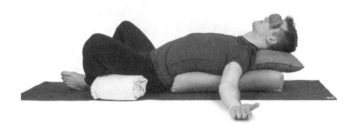

Props

- Bolster
- Pillow
- Two rolled blankets
- Eye pillow (optional)

Description

1. Place a bolster lengthwise on the mat, and place a pillow at the top of the bolster.
2. Sit in front of the bolster, leaving some space between the hips and the bolster. Bend the legs and bring the soles of the feet together, tucking the heels in close to the body.
3. Place a rolled blanket beneath the upper thighs, and let the thighs release into the blankets. The height of the rolled blankets should support the weight of the thighs so there is no tension or pull felt at the inner groins. The height on each side should be the same.
4. Gently lie over the bolster so the length of the bolster supports the length of the spine and the pillow supports the head. The chin should tilt slightly downward so there is no tension at the back or front of the neck.
5. Roll the shoulder blades down the back, and let the arms rest comfortably by your sides.
6. For deeper relaxation, place an eye pillow over the eyes.

Supported Bridge

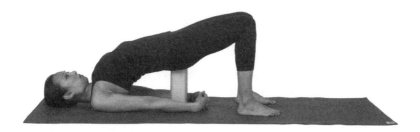

Prop

- Yoga block

Description

1. Start lying supine with the legs bent and the feet flat on the floor, parallel and hip-distance apart.

2. Press into the feet and raise the hips. Place a yoga block at the sacrum, allowing it to rest on the block. Place the block at a height suitable for the body, eventually placing it at its highest height.

3. Lengthen the tailbone and pubic bone toward the legs. The tops of the shoulders rest on the floor.

4. Roll the shoulder blades down the back and extend the arms. Alternatively, you can clasp the hands beneath you and extend them toward the feet.

5. Raise the chin slightly to elongate the back of the neck.

6. Continue to press into the inner feet to keep the knees from splaying.

Supported Forward Bend

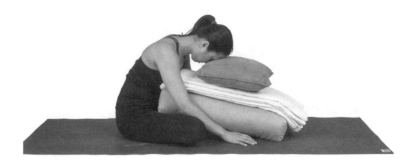

Props

- Bolster
- One or two folded blankets
- Two rolled blankets (optional)
- Two pillows

Description

1. Start in a simple cross-legged seated position. Experiment with moving the feet closer or farther from the body to find a comfortable placement for the hips and thighs, ensuring there is no discomfort in the knees.
2. Place the bolster on the thighs with the narrow end close to the body. Place one or two blankets or two pillows over the bolster. You will have to experiment to find the height of support most suitable for your body.
3. Moving from the hips, come into a forward bend and rest the upper body on the support.
4. Place the hands beneath the forehead for support, or let them rest on the floor beside you. Drop the chin slightly to lengthen the back of the neck. The head should not drop below the shoulders.
5. After half the time has passed, lift out of the forward bend, change the crossing of the legs, and return to the supported forward bend.
6. If the outer ankles pressing into the floor are painful, place a folded towel beneath them.
7. If the knees are quite high off the ground, place a rolled blanket under each thigh. Be sure the knees are completely pain free.

Variation

1. Although more challenging, this pose can also be done with the legs straight and wide. In this case, the bolster support rests on the floor. With this variation you may need more height.

Supported Child's Pose

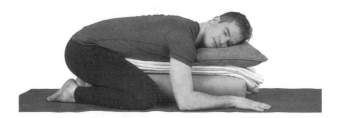

Props

- Bolster
- One or two folded blankets
- Two pillows (optional)

Description

1. Start on hands and knees on a yoga mat with the big toes together and the knees apart. Start with the knees at hip distance and move them farther apart to suit your body.

2. If the knees hurt, place a folded blanket beneath them.

3. Place one or two folded blankets over the bolster. Place the narrow end of the bolster between the inner thighs and move into child's pose (see chapter 7) by sitting back on the heels and extending the upper body forward, letting the chest and abdomen rest on the support.

4. Keep the hips on the heels and lengthen the upper body. If you feel excessive tugging around the knees, place a pillow between the heels and the hips.

5. Rest the head to one side; after half the time has passed, switch to the other side.

6. Let the arms rest comfortably over the support or by your sides.

Legs Up the Wall

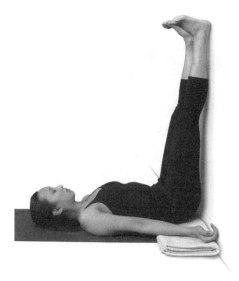

Props

- Bolster or folded blanket
- Eye pillow (optional)

Description

1. Place the yoga mat with the narrow edge touching the wall.
2. Place the blanket at the bottom edge of the mat, also touching the wall.
3. Sit on the blanket with the legs bent and one hip touching the wall.
4. Rotate the upper body and hips to bring both sitting bones toward the wall and the upper body to the mat. The upper body is on the mat, and the legs are up the wall with the hips on the blanket and as close to the wall as possible.
5. Straighten the legs and let the arms rest comfortably by your sides.
6. The support provides added comfort and release for the lower back. However, the pose can also be done with no support with the hips simply resting on the floor.
7. Relax the weight of the legs into the wall and that of the upper body to the floor. If you feel a deep hamstrings stretch, bend the legs slightly.
8. Note that getting into this pose may be awkward at first. Experiment with the positioning of the blanket, and you will soon find a way to move into this pose with ease.
9. For deeper relaxation, place the eye pillow over the eyes.

Chapter 12

Yoga Sequences

It's time to get to your yoga mat and let the magic unfold. This chapter outlines a number of sequences of various lengths and degrees of challenge. Read the descriptions and start with one that suits you. Change it up, though, and try some of the others. Some poses appear in many of the sequences. The sequences emphasize the hips, hamstrings, and spine because these are especially beneficial for the potential trouble zones for runners.

Yoga poses, or asanas, are generally categorized into the following types: sitting, standing, forward bends, back bends, twists, inversions, and reclining. Each type of yoga pose has its own unique purpose and benefit. The sequence in which you complete the yoga poses is also important; general warm-up; active strength building or specific body focus; cool-down and savasana. Remember that breathing is an integral part of your physical yoga practice, as described in chapter 3. Be sure to begin your yoga practice with a few rounds of full, deep yogic breathing. As with any new exercise routine, consult your doctor first.

Practice Guidelines

The following guidelines will help you get the most out of your yoga practice:

- Practice yoga on an empty stomach.
- Make sure the room temperature is warm to hot, as desired. Practicing in a cold room is less than desirable.
- Wear comfortable clothing; most running attire is fine.
- Practice in bare feet.
- Invest in a good-quality yoga mat. A yoga mat should stick to the floor and provide firm cushioning and a safe, nonsliding surface for the hands and feet.

- If you plan to use props, have them within easy reach.

- Do not be surprised if you sweat during a yoga practice; in fact, you should welcome sweating because it indicates that you are generating internal heat. If your mat becomes wet from sweating, try using a yoga towel, which absorbs sweat and sticks to the mat.

- Unless otherwise specified, hold poses for 5 breaths in the sequences laid out. Of course, if you are in a pose that feels particularly beneficial, you can hold for longer. Likewise, as you gain strength and stability, you can lengthen the holding time to 10 breaths. There is no universal rule about holding times in yoga, so feel free to experiment and choose times that suit you.

- Muscular and joint imbalances will become evident as a result of your yoga practice, and you may notice that one side is more open, tighter, weaker, or stronger. Whatever variation of the pose you do on one side you should do on the other side. Maintaining symmetry in the poses will help your body become symmetrical. This includes holding the poses for an equal number of breaths on each side. However, if you notice a considerable difference between sides in a particular pose, you can hold the tighter, more restricted side longer or do it twice.

- Listen to your body and never push through pain. Learn to differentiate between a stretch pain and a red alert pain, and avoid the latter. Never apply the adage "No pain, no gain!"

- The greatest benefits come from a regular yoga practice: several times per week with practices of varied duration. Do not try to make up missed yoga sessions by doing one superlong or superhard practice. If your practice becomes derailed, ease back into it slowly.

- Do not measure improvement in your poses. A regular practice will lead to deep changes in your body, some more evident than others. Keep in mind that the benefits compound over time, and enjoy the feeling you have after each practice.

- Save your competitive streak for the track! Yoga is not a competitive sport (with yourself or with others). Rather, view it as a time to simply be with yourself and put your expectations aside.

- Have fun! Experiment and add variety to your practice. As you attempt challenging poses, do so with an attitude of fun.

- Make savasana the last pose of every yoga practice. Even just a few moments lying still in body and mind will help you assimilate the energy from your practice. Plus, it just feels good!

ESSENTIAL SEQUENCES

This section provides yoga sequences for all occasions. They are varied in length and degree of challenge, and even include a series of exercises that can be done while watching TV. Because the greatest benefits are gained from practicing frequently and consistently, and respecting that time is a factor, a few short sequences that are easy to incorporate after every run have been included. However, to get the deeper benefits related to strength and flexibility, we have included longer sequences as well.

In these sequences, the recommended holding time for each pose is five breaths, unless otherwise indicated. Exceptions are the sun salutations, in which each pose is held for either an inhale or an exhale before remaining in downward dog for 5 breaths. Some poses are held for a shorter time, because they are intended to be brief transitions, and some are held for longer to build strength and stamina.

In many cases there are a number of ways to come into or out of a pose, For example, if the pose is being done from standing, you simply move the feet apart to the indicated distance. However, if the pose is being done as part of a flowing sequence, you may be instructed to move into the pose from downward dog. The set-up and alignment remains the same once you are in the pose.

Often a pose is done on one side and then the other. In some of the sequences, a series of three or four poses are completed on one side and then the other. This style of sequencing is more challenging but builds greater strength and improves focus and concentration. In the same way that you continue to run even when you are tired, stay with the poses when your mind says otherwise, and always return to the breath.

Sequence 1: TV Yoga

This sequence can be done apart from your scheduled yoga practice time. Called TV yoga, the exercises can be done while watching your favorite program or the nightly news and are an effective way to gain the benefits of yoga on an ongoing basis. Do as many as you have time for, and repeat as many times as you wish.

Plantar massage (p. 62)		• Roll along the entire length of the foot, from each joint to the heel. Repeat each segment up to 3 times.
Quadriceps and iliotibial band rollouts (p. 74)		• Roll at least 10 times on each side and for each variation.
Hero pose (p. 64)		• Remain in this pose as long as there is no pain at the knees and ankles. If your feet start tingling or falling asleep, come out of the pose.
Toe spreading (p. 66)		• Hold for 5 to 10 breaths on each side.
Hero toes (p. 65)		• Hold for 5 breaths, return to hero pose, and repeat up to 3 times.
Cow pose, shoulder stretch (p. 123)		• Hold each side for 5 breaths. • This pose can be done while seated in hero pose or hero, seated in simple cross leg (alternate the cross of the legs when changing arm position), or standing.
Bound angle (p. 162)		• Hold for 10 breaths.

Sequence 2: No Excuses Post-Run (5 to 8 Minutes)

Fitting everything into your daily schedule is challenging, so it is easy to conclude that you cannot add one more thing. However, it doesn't get easier than this; you can do this sequence with your running shoes on in as little as 5 minutes. This is a mandatory sequence, so make it a habit after every run.

Equal standing, arms overhead (p. 84)		• Hold for 5 breaths. • Place feet hip-distance apart.
Standing side bend (p. 85)		• Bend to the right; hold for 5 breaths. • Repeat on the other side.
Half downward dog (p. 86)		• Hold for 5 to 10 breaths. • Repeat 2 or 3 times. • If a wall is not available, use a tree, ledge, or tabletop.
Knee to ankle balance (p. 157)		• Hold for 5 breaths on each side.
Squat (p. 161)		• Hold for 5 to 10 breaths.

Sequence 3: Runners' Hot Spots (10 to 15 Minutes)

This sequence is a short yoga practice for runners' most common problem areas: the hips, hamstrings, and lower back. It is a relatively simple sequence suitable for both beginners and those with yoga experience. Included are some fundamental yoga poses that stretch and strengthen the spine, stretch the hips and hamstrings, and build upper-body strength (through holding downward dog a number of times). This sequence introduces a flow: One pose leads to the next in a continuous flow of movement and breath.

Child's pose (p. 88)		• Hold for 5 to 10 breaths. • Press into the hands and knees, lift the belly, and come to tabletop position on the hands and knees, with shoulders over the wrists, knees over the hips, and toes pointed.
Cat–dog stretch (p. 87)		• Start in neutral spinal position. Alternate movements for 5 full breaths. • Return the spine to neutral. • Place the hands at the front of the mat and slide knees back so they are behind the hips. • Curl toes under and lift the hips.
Downward dog (p. 89)		• Hold for 5 breaths.
Standing wide-leg forward bend (p. 136)		• From downward dog, step the right foot to the right hand, turn the right toes inward, and bring the feet to parallel. • Walk the hands and upper body to the left so that the hands are under the shoulders, with the arms and legs straight. • Press into the palms, lengthen the sides of the torso, and extend the breastbone forward to lengthen the spine. • Hold for 5 breaths. • Pivot on the toes of the left foot, turn the right toes forward, walk the hands to either side of the right foot, slide the right leg back, and return to downward dog.

Downward dog (p. 89)		• Hold for 5 breaths. • Slide the right knee to the right hand.
Pigeon (p. 159)		• Hold for 5 breaths. • Press into the hands, lift the hips, and return to downward dog. • Repeat on the other side. • If one side is markedly tighter, hold it for 10 breaths.
Downward dog (p. 89)		• Hold for 5 breaths. • Step the right foot to the right hand.
Low lunge (p. 164)		• Hold each side for 5 breaths.
Downward dog (p. 89)		• Hold for 5 breaths. • Step both feet forward to the hands, come to sitting, and lie supine.
Bridge (p. 121)		• Hold for 5 to 10 breaths. • Slowly lower hips to the floor.
Thighs to chest (p. 92)		• Slowly roll the hips from side to side while taking 5 breaths.
Supine twist (p. 93)		• Hold each side for 5 breaths.
Savasana (corpse pose) (p. 97)		• Hold for at least 2 minutes.

Sequence 4: Weekly Overall Tune-Up (60 to 75 Minutes)

Sun salutations are a series of poses that are linked by breath. The breath and movement are coordinated and they warm up the body by stretching and contracting many of the body's main muscles. Through the movement phase, the poses are held for only an inhale or an exhale and typically the last pose, downward dog, is held for 5 breaths.

Because of the flow of movement, sun salutations get the blood pumping and distribute energy (prana) throughout the body, in addition to creating internal heat in preparation for the remainder of the practice. There are many sun salutation variations; the style and variations in these sequences strengthen the entire body. They are especially great for building upper-body and core strength. Although initially they may be quite challenging, if you follow the alignment details and practice them on a regular basis, you will notice a remarkable gain in your strength, flexibility . . . and your running!

This specific sequence improves overall balance and symmetry in the body as it works on virtually all of the major muscles and joints. The sequence starts with a brief warm-up before a more intense working phase and ends with some seated and supine poses for the cool-down phase. If you have enough energy after a run, this is a great way to actively recover. Like a car that has been tuned up, your body will hum! Figure 12.1 illustrates one complete sun salutation. For an adequate warm-up, do at least 3 complete sun salutations and build to 5 to 8. If you are feeling strong and energetic, do more. It is important to listen to your body.

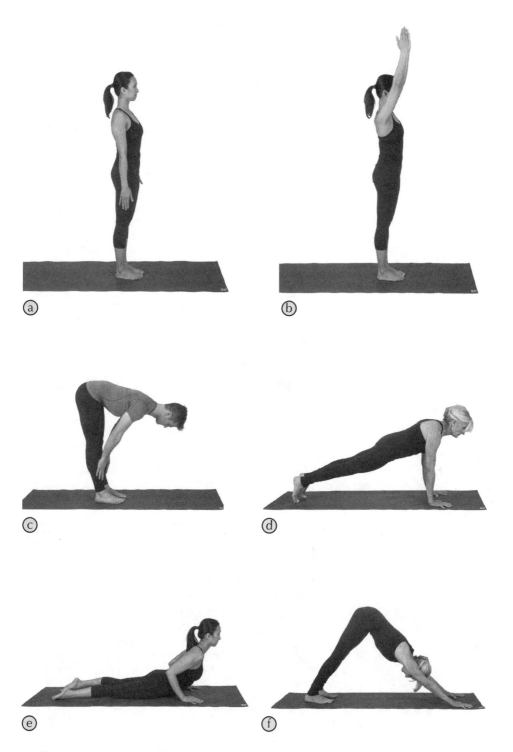

▶ **Figure 12.1** Sun salutation I.

Sequence 4: Weekly Overall Tune-Up

Hero pose (p. 64)		• Hold for 10 breaths. If painful, start with fewer breaths and build up to 10 over time.
Hero toes (p. 65)		• Hold for 10 breaths. If painful, start with fewer breaths and build up to 10 over time. • Place the hands at the front of the mat and come to downward dog.
Downward dog (p. 89)		• Hold for 5 to 10 breaths. • Inhale, press the hands into the floor, lift the belly, step both feet forward, and come into equal standing.
Sun Salutation I The next six poses comprise one sun salutation. Complete 3 to 8 sun salutations, and after your final one, remain in downward dog.		
Equal standing (p. 61)		• Hold for 3 deep, even breaths.
Equal standing, arms overhead (p. 84)		• Inhale and raise the arms overhead.
Standing forward bend (p. 132)		• Exhale, hinging from the hips, and fold into a forward bend. • Place the hands at the front of the mat, bending the legs if necessary, and strongly pull in the belly. • Step the feet back.
Plank (p. 113)		• Hold for 5 to 10 breaths. • Exhale, release the knees to the floor, and lower the upper body to the floor. Pull the belly and front of the ribs in so the lower back does not sag.
Cobra (p. 95)		• Inhale to lift the chest and hold for 3 breaths. • Exhale to lower chest to the floor. • Inhale, press hands into the floor, lift to the knees, and lift hips to move into downward dog.

Downward dog (p. 89)		• Hold for 5 breaths. • Inhale. Press the hands to the floor, lift the belly, and step the feet forward. • After your final sun salutation, inhale and step the right foot forward for lunges.
Complete the next two poses on the right side first, return to downward dog, and then repeat on the left side.		
Low lunge (p. 164)		• Hold for 5 breaths. • Move into lunge twist.
Lunge twist (p. 166)		• Hold for 5 breaths. • Step front foot back. • Return to downward dog.
Downward dog (p. 89)		• Hold for 5 breaths. • Step the right foot forward and release the left knee to the floor.
Complete the next two poses on the right side first, return to downward dog, and then repeat on the left side.		
Kneeling lunge (p. 164)		• Hold for 5 breaths. • Slide the right leg to the right, aligning the heel of the right foot with the left knee for gate pose.
Gate (p. 137)		• Hold for 5 breaths. • After completing the second side, slide the front leg back, place the hands on the floor, and return to downward dog.
Downward dog (p. 89)		• Hold for 5 breaths.

(continued)

Sequence 4: Weekly Overall Tune-Up *(continued)*

Complete the next three poses on the right side first, return to downward dog, and then repeat on the left side.

High lunge (p. 164)		• Hold for 5 breaths. • Without changing the position of the legs, place the left hand to the floor, twisting the torso to the left for lunge twist.
Lunge twist (p. 166)		• Hold for 5 breaths. • Return both hands to the floor then lift the torso upright and return to high lunge.
High lunge (p. 164)		• Hold for 3 breaths. • Take the hands to the floor and step the right foot back to return to downward dog.
Downward dog (p. 89)		• Hold for 5 breaths. • Slide the right knee to the right hand.
Pigeon (p. 159)		• Hold each side for 5 to 10 breaths.
Downward dog (p. 89)		• Hold for 5 breaths. • Step both feet forward.
Equal standing (p. 61)		• Hold for 1 breath.

Complete the next two poses on the right side first, followed by the left side.

Straight-leg lunge (p. 134)		• Note that the back foot is angled and the heel is on the floor. • Hold for 5 breaths.
Revolved triangle (p. 135)		• Hold for 5 breaths. • Return to equal standing, switch the legs, and repeat the 2 poses on the other side.
Equal standing (p. 61)		• Hold for 1 breath.

Complete the next two poses on the right side first, followed by the left side.

Warrior II (p. 154)		• Hold for 5 breaths.
Extended side stretch (p. 152)		• Hold for 5 breaths. • Repeat the two poses on the other side.
Equal standing (p. 61)		• Hold for 1 breath.
Simple balance (p. 63)		• Hold for 5 breaths on each side.

(continued)

Sequence 4: Weekly Overall Tune-Up *(continued)*

Tree (p. 158)		• Hold for 5 breaths on each side.
Equal standing (p. 61)		• Hold for 1 breath. • Place feet slightly wider than hip distance.
Squat (p. 161)		• Hold for 5 breaths. • Place the hands on the floor, sit, and straighten the legs.
Staff pose (p. 90)		• Hold for 5 breaths.
Double pigeon (p. 160)		• Hold for 5 breaths on each side. • Straighten the legs and return to staff pose.
Bound angle (p. 162)		• Hold for 5 to 10 breaths. • Straighten the legs.
Simple seated twist (p. 91)		• Hold for 5 breaths on each side. • Straighten the legs and return to staff pose. • Cross the legs into a simple cross-leg position.
Cow pose, shoulder stretch (p. 123)		• Hold for 5 breaths. • Change the cross of the legs and arm position and repeat on the other side. • Hold for 5 breaths. • Straighten the legs and lie supine.

Supine hamstrings stretch (p. 140)		• Hold each side of the three parts of this pose for 5 breaths. • Repeat on the other side. • Bring both legs to the floor and bend the legs.
Bridge (p. 121)		• Hold for 5 to 10 breaths.
Thighs to chest (p. 92)		• Hold for 5 breaths. • Straighten and extend the legs.
Savasana (corpse pose) (p. 97)		• Remain in this pose for 5 minutes.

Sequence 5: Strength and Stamina (75 to 90 minutes)

This is the most challenging of the sequences in this book. It is a powerful sequence that builds strength and flexibility in the upper body, core, and legs. Yoga experience is required; you should be able to complete several of the sun salutations in sequence 4 with relative ease. This practice also builds stamina as you move from one pose to another with a continuous flow of breath. This is a perfect sequence for a day when you are not running. The sequence starts with abdominal work, which serves as an effective warm-up and reminder to continue using these muscles throughout the sequence.

This sequence includes a more challenging version of the sun salutations (sun salutation II), which includes additional poses for greater core and upper-body strengthening (see figure 12.2). As in sequence 4, many poses are held for only an inhale or an exhale through the movement phase; others are held for 5 breaths.

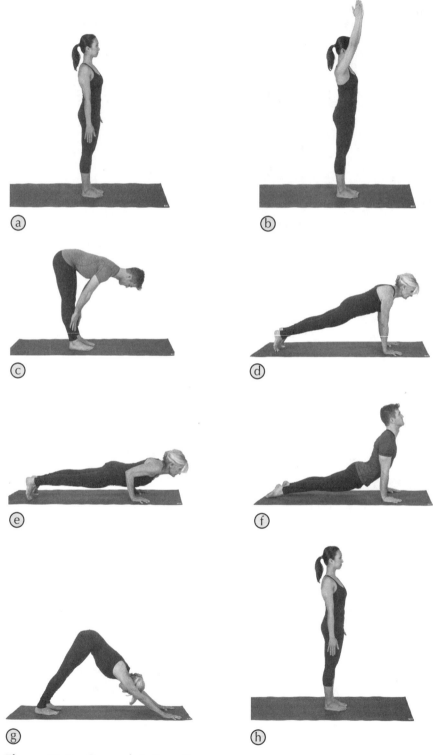

▶ **Figure 12.2** Sun salutation II.

Sequence 5: Strength and Stamina

Ab curls I (p. 111)		• Do 10 repetitions in one set, or stop when the hips start to sway and no longer stable. • Repeat up to 3 sets.
Ab curls II (p. 112)		• Do 10 repetitions in one set, or stop when the hips start to sway and are no longer stable. • Repeat up to 3 sets.
Sun Salutation II Complete sun salutation II (the following eight poses) 3 to 5 times. After the final sun salutation, remain in downward dog, then move into plank with the feet together, and then pivot to the right to move into side plank.		
Equal standing (p. 61)		• Take 1 full breath.
Equal standing, arms overhead (p. 84)		• Inhale and raise the arms overhead.
Standing forward bend (p. 132)		• Exhale, hinging from the hips, and fold into a forward bend. • Place the hands at the front of the mat, bend the legs if necessary, and strongly pull in the belly. • Exhale and step the feet back.
Plank (p. 113)		• Inhale. Note that it is fine to take a few breaths during these challenging poses if you need to. Do not hold your breath.
Chaturanga (yoga push-up) (p. 114)		• Exhale and slowly lower to the ground. • Point the toes back so the tops of the feet are on the floor.
Upward dog (p. 119)		• Inhale as you move into the pose. • Exhale, curl the toes under, lift the belly, and press the hips back into downward dog.

(continued)

Sequence 5: Strength and Stamina *(continued)*

Downward dog (p. 89)		• Hold for 5 breaths. • Inhale. Press the hands to the floor, lift the belly, and step the feet forward.
Equal standing (p. 61)		• Continue inhaling to equal standing. Exhale.
Side plank (p. 115)		• Hold for 5 breaths on each side, pivoting on the feet and returning to plank between sides. • After the second side, return to plank.
Plank (p. 113)		• Inhale; take an extra breath if needed.
Chaturanga **(yoga push-up)** (p. 114)		• Exhale to lower the body to the floor. • Point the toes back so the tops of the feet are on the floor. • Keep the elbows over the wrists.
Upward dog (p. 119)		• Inhale as you move into the pose. • Exhale, curl the toes under, lift the belly, and press the hips back to move into downward dog.
Downward dog (p. 89)		• Hold for 5 breaths. • Inhale. Press the hands into the floor, lift the belly, and step the feet forward.
Equal standing (p. 61)		• Continue inhaling to equal standing. Exhale.

Sun Salutation II
Repeat sun salutation II. From downward dog, move into dolphin.

Dolphin (downward dog variation) (p. 116)		• Hold for 5 breaths. • Keep the forearms firmly grounded and walk the feet back and lower the hips so they are in line with the upper body.
Dolphin plank (p. 117)		• Hold for 5 breaths. • Walk the feet forward and return to dolphin (downward dog variation); then straighten the arms and come into downward dog.
Downward dog (p. 89)		• Hold for 5 breaths. • Step the right foot forward to the right hand, and lower the left knee to the floor.
Kneeling lunge (p. 164)		• Hold each side for 5 breaths. • After the second side, step the front leg back and return to downward dog.
Downward dog (p. 89)		• Hold for 5 breaths. • Inhale. Step both feet forward and come to equal standing.

(continued)

Sequence 5: Strength and Stamina *(continued)*

Sun Salutation II

Repeat sun salutation II. From downward dog, step the right foot forward to the right hand for high lunge.

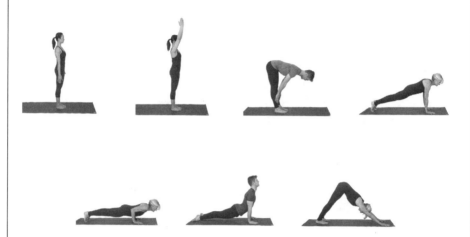

Do the next three poses on the right side; then return to downward dog and repeat on the left side.

High lunge (p. 164)		• Hold for 5 breaths. • Maintain the position of the legs and place the left hand on the floor, twisting the torso to the right for lunge twist.
Lunge twist (p. 166)		• Hold for 5 breaths. • Rest both hands on the floor, and lift the torso to return to high lunge.
High lunge (p. 164)		• Hold for 5 breaths. • Place the hands on the floor, and step the front leg back to return to downward dog.
Downward dog (p. 89)		• Hold for 5 breaths.

Complete the next two poses on the right side first, followed by the left side.		
Downward dog (leg extended variation) (p. 151)		• Hold for 5 breaths. • Strongly pull in the belly to raise the hips and step the right foot to the right hand.
High lunge (p. 164)		• Hold for 5 to 10 breaths. • Move the hands to the floor and step the leg back to return to downward dog. • Repeat on other side. • Step the front leg back and return to downward dog.
Downward dog (p. 89)		• Hold for 5 breaths.
Complete the next two poses on the right side, slide the front leg back to downward dog, and then repeat the two poses on the other side.		
Lizard (p. 167)		• Hold for 5 to 8 breaths on each side.
Twisted lizard (p. 168)		• Hold for 5 to 8 breaths on each side.
Downward dog (p. 89)		• Hold for 5 breaths.
Plank (p. 113)		• Hold for 1 breath.
Chaturanga (yoga push-up) (p. 114)		• Slowly lower to the ground.
Chest opener (p. 94)		• Hold for 5 breaths.
Half frog (p. 73)		• Hold for 5 to 8 breaths. • Repeat on the other side.

(continued)

Sequence 5: Strength and Stamina *(continued)*

Locust (p. 96)		• Hold for 3 to 5 breaths. • Repeat 5 times. • Between reps, release the head and legs to the floor, but keep the legs active with the tops of the feet pressing to the floor. • Press the hands to the floor, lift the upper body, bring the feet together with the knees apart, and come to child's pose.
Child's pose (p. 88)		• Hold for 5 to 10 breaths. Concentrate on expanding the lower back with each inhale. • Extend the arms to the front of the mat, press into the hands, lift the hips, and move into downward dog.
Downward dog (p. 89)		• Hold for 5 breaths. • Press the hands to the floor and step the feet forward.
Equal standing (p. 61)		• Hold for 1 breath.
Standing forward bend (p. 132)		• Hold for 5 breaths. • Place the hands in front of the feet on the floor, on blocks, or at the shins. • Return to equal standing.
Triangle (p. 133)		• Hold for 5 breaths on each side. • Return to equal standing.
Equal standing (p. 61)		• Hold for 1 breath.

Complete the next two poses on the right side first, return to equal standing, and then repeat on the left side.

Revolved triangle (p. 135)		• Hold for 5 breaths. • Return the torso to neutral and position it so it is parallel to the floor, with hands either resting on blocks or on the floor. • Come onto the toes of the back foot, and lift the leg parallel to the floor and in line with the hips for warrior III.
Warrior III (p. 156)		• Hold for 5 breaths. • Return the back leg to the floor.
Equal standing (p. 61)		• Hold for 1 breath.

Complete the next three poses on the right side, return to equal standing, and then repeat on the left side.

Warrior II (p. 154)		• Hold for 5 breaths. • Lean upper body to the right and rest the elbow on the knee for extended side stretch.
Extended side stretch (p. 152)		• Hold for 5 breaths.
Bound side stretch (p. 153)		• Hold for 5 breaths. • Press into the feet, lift upright, pivot on the feet, and repeat the three poses on the other side.
Equal standing (p. 61)		• Hold for 1 breath.
Standing Egyptian (p. 155)		• Repeat up to 3 sets of 5 breaths, but do not straighten the legs between sets. Varying the arm positions is optional.

(continued)

Sequence 5: Strength and Stamina *(continued)*

Equal standing (p. 61)		• Hold for 1 breath.
Knee to ankle balance (p. 157)		• Hold for 5 breaths on each side.

Sun Salutation II
Complete sun salutation II. Remain in downward dog for one breath, then move into pigeon.

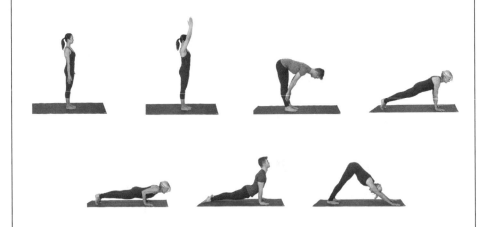

Pigeon (p. 159)		• Hold for 5 breaths on each side. • When coming out of the pose, slide the front leg back and come to downward dog.
Downward dog (p. 89)		• Remain in downward dog for 1 breath, step the feet forward, bend the legs, and sit
Staff pose (p. 90)		• Hold for 5 breaths.
Seated forward bend (p. 138)		• Hold for 5 breaths. • Return to staff pose.

Upward plank (p. 118)		• Lower the hips to the floor and return to staff pose.
Double pigeon (p. 160)		• Hold for 5 breaths on each side. • If the bottom knee is not on the ground, straighten the bottom leg.
Simple seated twist (p. 91)		• Hold for 5 breaths on each side. • Return to staff pose.
Seated wide-leg forward bend (p. 139)		• Hold for 5 breaths. • Bring the legs together and return to staff pose.
Bound angle (p. 162)		• Hold for 5 to 10 breaths. • Bring the knees together, straighten the legs, and return to staff pose.
Boat (p. 120)		• Hold for 5 breaths, then rest the feet on the floor and hug the thighs to the chest. • Repeat 5 times. • After the last one, release the feet to the floor and lie supine.
Supine hamstrings stretch (p. 140)		• Hold each side and variation for 5 breaths.
Bridge (p. 121)		• Hold for 5 to 10 breaths.
Thighs to chest (p. 92)		• Hold for 3 to 5 breaths.

(continued)

Sequence 5: Strength and Stamina *(continued)*

Supine twist (p. 93)		• Hold each side for 5 breaths.
Savasana (corpse pose) (p. 97)		• Remain in this pose for 5 minutes.

BODY PART–SPECIFIC SEQUENCES

As you embark on your yoga journey, you will develop a better understanding of your body's strengths, weaknesses, tight spots, and more limber areas. Over time, an overall body-balancing yoga practice will help to even out the marked imbalances. In addition, from time to time you can include a yoga practice that targets a specific area. Listening to and being in tune with the inner workings of your body may reveal an area that feels particularly tight or sore. When you notice this, you may want to practice the sequence for that body part for a few days and observe the results.

Although these sequences are excellent ways to deal with potential problem areas, they should be practiced only occasionally, as needed. They should not be used in place of the essential sequences. To restore your body to its desired state of balance and symmetry, your regular practice should include overall body work.

Sequence 6: Hips (45 to 60 Minutes)

This series of poses focuses on the hips and includes hip-strengthening and hip-opening poses. This sequence is beneficial for those recovering from injury, especially if the diagnosed problem relates to weak glutes or weak hips. Additionally, this is suitable for those times when the hips are feeling particularly tight or achy, perhaps following a heavy training schedule. This sequence is also helpful for those who have spent an inordinate amount of time seated, as when traveling in a car or airplane. For sun salutations in this sequence, use either sun salutation I or II.

Finding the gluteus medius (p. 145)		• Review the detailed description for how to locate and contract the gluteus medius. If this is difficult, practice several times. If you find this work easy, skip this step and move to the next pose.
Kneeling clam (p. 149)		• Repeat 10 times on each side.
Tabletop with leg extended (p. 150)		• Keep hips square by contracting outer left hip (gluteus medius) and pulse the right extended leg 10 times, keeping the leg straight and moving it up and down about 6 inches (15 cm). • Repeat on the other side. • Release both knees to the floor hip-distance apart, curl the toes under, lift the hips, and come into downward dog.
Downward dog (leg extended variation) (p. 151)		• Hold for 5 breaths on each side.

(continued)

Sequence 6: Hips *(continued)*

Complete sun salutation I or II three to five times for a warm-up. From last downward dog, step right foot forward for lunge.

Sun Salutation I

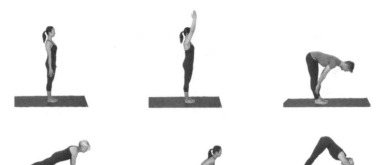

Sun Salutation II

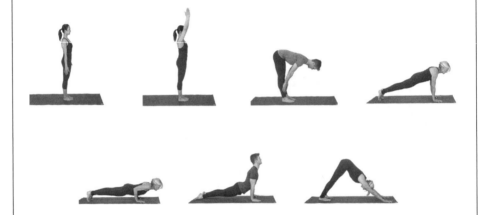

Low lunge (p. 164)		• Hold for 5 breaths on each side. • Return to downward dog.
Downward dog (p. 89)		• Hold for 3 to 5 breaths.
High lunge (p. 164)		• Hold for 5 breaths on each side.

Downward dog (p. 89)		• Hold for 3 to 5 breaths.
Repeat the next 2 poses on one side and then repeat on the other.		
Lizard (p. 167)		• Hold for 5 breaths.
Twisted lizard (p. 168)		• Hold for 5 to 8 breaths on each side. • Return to downward dog.
Downward dog (p. 89)		• Hold for 3 to 5 breaths.
High lunge (p. 164)		• Hold for 5 breaths on each side. • Bring the hands to the floor, slide the front leg back, and come to downward dog.
Downward dog (p. 89)		• Hold for 5 breaths. • Step the right foot forward so the right leg is at 90 degrees, release the left knee to the floor, and place a folded blanket beneath the knee.
Kneeling quadriceps stretch (p. 170)		• Hold for 10 breaths. As this pose gets easier, add variations, holding each one for 5 breaths. • Repeat on the other side. • Place hands on the floor, lift the hips, and come to downward dog.
Downward dog (p. 89)		• Hold for 5 breaths.

(continued)

Sequence 6: Hips *(continued)*

High lunge (p. 164)		• Hold for 10 breaths on each side. • After the quadriceps stretch, notice how the front groin of the back leg feels more spacious and open. • Bring the hands to the floor, step the front leg back, and come to downward dog.
Downward dog (p. 89)		• Hold for 3 to 5 breaths. • Step the feet forward and come to equal standing.
Equal standing (p. 61)		• Hold for 1 to 3 breath(s).
Repeat the next two poses on the right side first, and then repeat on the left side.		
Extended side stretch (p. 152)		• Hold for 5 breaths.
Bound side stretch (p. 153)		• Hold for 5 breaths.
Equal standing (p. 61)		• Hold for 1 breath.
Standing Egyptian (p. 155)		• Repeat up to 3 sets of 5 breaths, varying arm positions (as described in chapter 10). • Turn the toes in and straighten the legs. • Return to equal standing.

Complete one sun salutation, and from downward dog move into pigeon.

Sun Salutation I

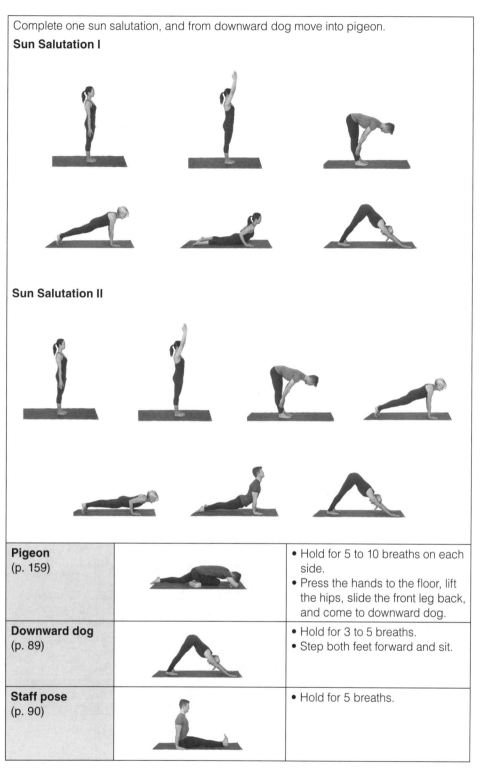

Sun Salutation II

Pigeon (p. 159)		• Hold for 5 to 10 breaths on each side. • Press the hands to the floor, lift the hips, slide the front leg back, and come to downward dog.
Downward dog (p. 89)		• Hold for 3 to 5 breaths. • Step both feet forward and sit.
Staff pose (p. 90)		• Hold for 5 breaths.

(continued)

Sequence 6: Hips *(continued)*

Double pigeon (p. 160)		• Hold for 5 breaths on each side.
Bound angle (p. 162)		• Hold for 10 breaths. • Bring the knees together, straighten the legs, and return to staff pose. Lie supine.
Internal rotator stretch (p. 163)		• Hold for 5 to 10 breaths on each side.
Thighs to chest (p. 92)		• Slowly roll the hips from side to side while taking 5 breaths.
Savasana (corpse pose) (p. 97)		• Remain in this pose for 5 minutes.

Sequence 7: Hamstrings (45 to 60 Minutes)

Whether from running or lifestyle habits, the hamstrings may require some additional attention from time to time. Be mindful of the messages your body sends, and when the hamstrings are feeling particularly tight, practice this sequence for a few days and observe the changes. This sequence focuses on stretching the hamstrings but also incorporates strengthening. This series of poses is helpful when recovering from a hamstring injury, but be particularly mindful of not overstretching. For sun salutations in this sequence, use either sun salutation I or II.

Hamstrings eccentric stretch (p. 130)		• This is a gentle and safe way to stretch the hamstrings with a reduced risk of over stretching. • Hold each side for 10 breaths. • Roll onto the belly, press the hands to the floor, and come to hands and knees.
Hamstrings curl (p. 131)		• Repeat the pulsing action 10 times, keeping the entire length of the hamstrings contracted. • Repeat on the other side. • Option: Complete up to 3 sets (10 pulses per set).

Complete sun salutation I or II three to five times for an overall body warm-up. From last downward dog, step right foot to the right hand.

Sun Salutation I

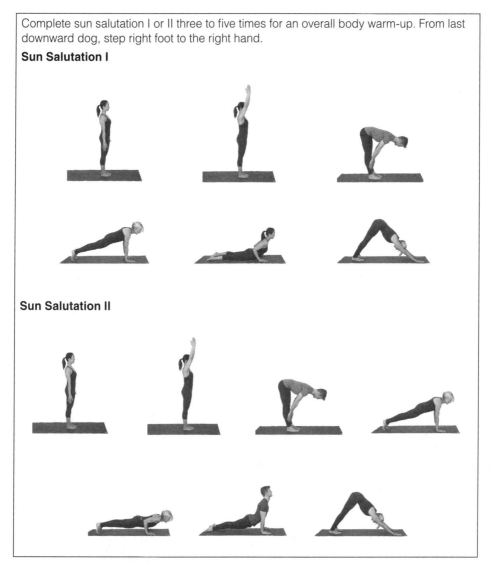

Sun Salutation II

(continued)

Sequence 7: Hamstrings *(continued)*

Complete the next three poses on one side, return to downward dog, and repeat on the other side.		
Straight-leg lunge (p. 134)		• Stay on the toes on the back foot and keep the hips square. • Hold for 5 breaths. • Bend the back leg and release the knee to the floor. Be sure the front leg is at 90 degrees.
Kneeling lunge (p. 164)		• Hold for 5 breaths. • Slide the left leg to the left, aligning the foot with the right knee.
Gate (p. 137)		• Hold for 5 breaths.
Downward dog (p. 89)		• Hold for 5 breaths. • Step both feet forward.
Equal standing (p. 61)		• Hold for 1 to 3 breaths.
Revolved triangle (p. 135)		• Hold for 5 breaths on each side.
Warrior III (p. 156)		• Hold for 5 breaths on each side.
Equal standing (p. 61)		• Hold for 1 breath.

Triangle (p. 133)		• Hold for 5 breaths on each side.
Equal standing (p. 61)		• Hold for 1 breath.
Standing wide-leg forward bend (p. 136)		• Hold for 5 to 10 breaths.
Equal standing (p. 61)		• Hold for 1 breath. • Squat and sit.

Sun Salutation I

Complete the first four poses from sun salutation I. From plank, slowly release your body to the floor and lie prone.

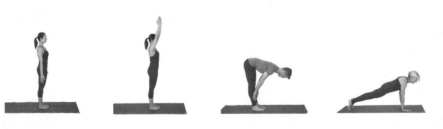

Half frog (p. 73)		• Hold for 8 to 10 breaths. Repeat on other side.
Locust (p. 96)		• If lifting both legs, hold for 5 breaths. If lifting one leg at a time, hold for 5 breaths on each side. Focus on keeping the hamstrings contracted. • Repeat 3 sets. • Press into the hands and knees, curl the toes under, lift the hips, and come into downward dog. • Option: Come to child's pose (see chapter 7).

(continued)

Sequence 7: Hamstrings *(continued)*

Downward dog (p. 89)		• Hold for 5 to 10 breaths. • Step the feet forward, squat, and sit.
Staff pose (p. 90)		• Hold for 5 breaths.
Seated forward bend (p. 138)		• Hold for 5 to 10 breaths.
Seated wide-leg forward bend (p. 139)		• Hold for 5 breaths. • Bring the legs together and lie supine.
Supine hamstrings stretch (p. 140)		• Hold each side and variation for 5 breaths.
Bridge (p. 121)		• Hold for 5 breaths. • Repeat 2 to 4 times.
Thighs to chest (p. 92)		• Hold for 5 breaths. • Slowly roll the hips from side to side.
Savasana (corpse pose) (p. 97)		• Remain in this pose for 5 minutes.

Sequence 8: Back (45 to 60 Minutes)

This sequence focuses on movements of the spine, including stretching, strengthening, and rejuvenating twists. This is a suitable sequence to include when you are experiencing back pain or more stiffness than usual. Note that this sequence is not flowing. Simply set up for each pose as instructed and move to the next one. In addition to these poses, strengthening the abdominals is helpful for the back, so regularly practice sequences 4 and 5.

Cat–dog stretch (p. 87)		• Start in neutral spine position. Alternate movements for 5 full breaths. • Return the spine to neutral. • Press the hips back toward the heels, and come into child's pose.
Child's pose (p. 88)		• Hold for 5 deep breaths, feeling the lower back expand with the inhale. • Roll onto your back.
Ab curls I (p. 111)		• Complete 10 repetitions for 1 set. Pause and take 3 deep breaths. Perform up to 5 sets. • Bring the feet to the floor with the legs bent, knees together, and feet hip-distance apart. Take 5 deep abdominal breaths (see chapter 3 for description), letting the belly expand and release with every breath.
Ab curls II (p. 112)		• Complete 10 repetitions for 1 set. Pause and take 3 deep breaths. Perform up to 5 sets. • Bring the feet to the floor with the legs bent, knees together, and feet hip-distance apart. Take 5 deep abdominal breaths (see chapter 3 for description), letting the belly expand and release with every breath.

(continued)

Sequence 8: Back *(continued)*

Half downward dog (p. 86)		• Hold for 10 breaths.
Child's pose (p. 88)		• Hold for 5 deep breaths, feeling the lower back expand with the inhale. • Curl the toes under, lift the hips, and come into downward dog.
Downward dog (p. 89)		• Hold for 5 to 10 breaths. • Release the knees and upper body to the floor and lie prone.
Chest opener (p. 94)		• Hold for 5 breaths. Release and take 2 breaths. • Repeat 3 times.
Cobra (p. 95)		• Hold for 5 breaths. Release and take 2 breaths. • Repeat 3 times.
Locust (p. 96)		• Hold for 5 breaths. Release and take 2 breaths. • Repeat 3 times. • Press the hands and knees to the floor, lift the hips, and move into child's pose.
Child's pose (p. 88)		• Hold for 5 breaths. • Press the hands to the floor at the front of the mat, curl the toes under, and lift the hips to downward dog.
Downward dog (p. 89)		• Hold for 5 to 10 breaths. • Step the feet to the hands, squat, and sit.
Staff pose (p. 90)		• Hold for 5 breaths.
Simple seated twist (p. 91)		• Hold for 5 to 10 breaths on each side. • Return to staff pose and lie supine.

Thighs to chest (p. 92)		• Hold for 5 breaths. • Slowly roll the hips from side to side.
Supine twist (p. 93)		• Hold each side for 5 breaths.
Legs up the wall (p. 182)		• Place a bolster or folded blanket beneath the hips. • Hold for 5-10 minutes.
Savasana (corpse pose) (p. 97)		• Place a bolster or two folded blankets of even height beneath the knees. • Remain in this pose for 5 minutes.

Sequence 9: Knees (30 to 40 Minutes)

This sequence focuses on balancing the strength and flexibility of the quadriceps. You should do this sequence regularly if you have knee issues, but note that eventually you should incorporate it mindfully into your overall yoga practice.

Quadriceps and iliotibial band rollouts (p. 74)		• Roll the length of the quads and outer thighs 10 times each. • This may be very painful at the beginning, so use a leg position that is tolerable. • Move to the next degree of intensity as you are able to.
Plantar massage (p. 62)		• Hold the static pressing of the foot into the ball for 5 to 10 breaths. • Roll the sole of the foot over the ball, from each toe joint to the heel.

(continued)

Sequence 9: Knees *(continued)*

Hero pose (p. 64)		• Start by holding for 5 breaths and build up to several minutes. It is OK to come out of the pose; stretch out the legs, ankles, and feet; and then go back into it. • Use appropriate props so there is no intense pain in this pose. Build the length of time gradually and remove the props when appropriate.
Wall squat (p. 72)		• Start with a 1-minute hold and build up to 3 minutes. • It is imperative that the knees are over the ankles, the feet are parallel, and the toes face front.
Half frog (p. 73)		• Hold for 10 breaths on each side.
Equal standing (p. 61)		• Hold for 3 breaths, concentrating on contracting the inner quads.
Standing forward bend (p. 132)		• Step feet apart to hip distance and hinge from the hips into a forward bend, keeping the quadriceps contracted. • Hold for 5 breaths. • Press the palms into the floor, step the feet back, and move into downward dog.
Downward dog (p. 89)		• Hold for 5 to 10 breaths. • Contract the quadriceps as in equal standing. • Step the right foot forward to move into high lunge.
High lunge (p. 164)		• Alignment of the front leg should be as in wall squat. • Hold for 10 breaths, place the hands on the floor, slide the front leg back, and return to downward dog. • Repeat on the other side.

Downward dog (p. 89)		• Hold for 5 breaths. • Step both feet forward.
Equal standing (p. 61)		• Hold for 1 breath.
Repeat the next two poses on the right side first, followed by the left side.		
Warrior II (p. 154)		• Hold for 10 breaths. • Rest the right elbow on the right knee.
Extended side stretch (p. 152)		• Hold for 5 breaths. • Press into the feet, lift the torso, and pivot the feet to repeat the poses on the other side.
Equal standing (p. 61)		• Hold for 1 breath. • Squat, sit, and lie supine.
Hamstrings eccentric stretch (p. 130)		• Hold each side for 10 breaths.
Bridge (p. 121)		• Hold for 10 breaths.
Thighs to chest (p. 92)		• Hold for 5 breaths. • Slowly roll the hips from side to side.
Savasana (corpse pose) (p. 97)		• Remain in this pose for 2 to 3 minutes.

Sequence 10: Upper Body
(30 to 40 Minutes)

This sequence is for times when the upper body, including the neck and shoulders, is screaming with tension and tightness. This sequence reduces upper-body stress and strain. In addition to stretching out the tight areas, you must strengthen the muscles that support the upper body to reduce the chronic strain on the overused muscles. This series of poses includes both upper-body strengthening and stretching. Do this sequence when needed, but also include it in your overall yoga practice.

Equal standing (p. 61)		• Roll the upper arm bones back, slide the shoulder blades down the back, and lift the breastbone. • Hold for 5 breaths.
Eagle arms (p. 124)		• Hold for 5 breaths on each side. • Note: Pose can be done while standing.
Equal standing, arms overhead (p. 84)		• Hold for 5 breaths. Concentrate on keeping the shoulder blades down the back as you raise the arms.
Standing side bend (p. 85)		• Hold for 5 breaths. • Repeat on the other side.
Standing forward bend (p. 132)		• Hold for 5 breaths. • Bend the legs, place the hands on the floor shoulder-distance apart, press the hands into the floor, press the shoulder blades down the back, and step the feet back.
Downward dog (p. 89)		• Hold for 5 breaths. • The space from the base of the neck to the top of the arms should be soft and tension free.

Child's pose (p. 88)		• Hold for 5 breaths. • Wrap the arms around the thighs so that the shoulders are completely relaxed. • Extend the arms and place the hands at the front of the mat, shoulder-distance apart. Press into the hands, lift the hips, and curl the toes under.
Downward dog (p. 89)		• Hold for 5 breaths.
Dolphin (downward dog variation) (p. 116)		• Hold for 5 to 10 breaths. • Walk the feet back and lower the hips.
Dolphin plank (p. 117)		• Hold for 5 breaths. • Release the knees to the floor.
Child's pose (p. 88)		• Relax the upper body and hold for 5 breaths.
As these poses become less arduous, repeat the downward dog, dolphin, dolphin plank, and child's pose sequence 3 to 5 times.		
Downward dog (p. 89)		• Hold for 5 breaths. • Release the knees and torso to the floor.
Chest opener (p. 94)		• Hold for 5 breaths. Release and take 2 breaths. • Repeat 3 times.
Cobra (p. 95)		• Hold for 5 breaths. Release and take 2 breaths. • Repeat 3 times.
Upward dog (p. 119)		• Hold for 3 to 5 breaths. • Concentrate on keeping the shoulder blades down the back and the chest open.
Child's pose (p. 88)		• Hold for 5 breaths. • Wrap the arms around the thighs to release the shoulders. • Extend the arms to the front of the mat, curl the toes under, and lift the hips.

(continued)

Sequence 10: Upper Body *(continued)*

Downward dog (p. 89)		• Hold for 5 breaths. • Step both feet forward, squat, and sit.
Staff pose (p. 90)		• Hold for 5 breaths.
Upward plank (p. 118)		• Lower the hips to the floor and return to staff pose.
Staff pose (p. 90)		• Hold for one breath and cross the legs into a simple cross-leg or in hero pose.
Cow pose, shoulder stretch (p. 123)		• Hold for 5 breaths. • Change the cross of the legs and repeat on the other side.
Ear to shoulder (p. 122)		• Sit either in simple cross leg or in hero pose (see chapter 6 for detailed description). • Hold for 5 to 10 breaths on each side. • If sitting in simple cross leg, change the cross of the legs after the first side.
Bridge (p. 121)		• Hold for 10 breaths. • Option: Replace this pose with supported chest opener (see chapter 11).
Supine twist (p. 93)		• Hold for 5 breaths on each side. • As you move the legs to one side, press the opposite shoulder toward the floor.
Savasana (corpse pose) (p. 97)		• Remain in this pose for 2 to 3 minutes.

Chapter 13

Yoga Off the Mat

After a few yoga classes, many students comment on their heightened body awareness throughout the day and while running. Tightness in the neck, shoulders, and upper and lower back may have become ingrained in your body, and you have learned to live with the related discomfort. A regular yoga practice, with proper attention to detail, can relieve many of these chronic conditions. To accelerate the process, you can incorporate some easy exercises and simple reminders into your daily routines. These exercises are particularly beneficial to combat the effects of repetitive strain if you spend extended hours seated, whether in front of a computer or driving, or stand all day.

This chapter outlines some simple things that, done daily, will compound the benefits of yoga; basically, we are taking some fundamental yoga principles and applying them off the mat. These simple exercises will counter any bad habits and eventually ingrain good habits in your body.

Taking your yoga practice off the mat will result in better alignment while sitting, standing, and running. Not only will you look and feel better, but also some chronic aches and pains will subside and the benefits of your regular practice will compound.

As discussed in chapter 4, yoga is a mind–body discipline, inviting you to be present and in the moment when you practice. The mindfulness that you engage in on the yoga mat can also be applied to many of your daily tasks, reducing the boredom associated with some of these tasks and opening your eyes to things around you that often blur into the background. For example, when viewed as a chore, walking your dog may involve a quick dash outdoors, hoping the dog will complete his or her business quickly so you can get back to a more pressing demand. But walking the dog can be an opportunity to enjoy time with your best friend, take in the local landscape, see the neighbor's budding flowers, make eye contact and say hello to a passerby, or simply listen to the sound of your breath. The mundane can become joyful when approached with mindfulness.

The most powerful aspect of yoga is not what you do or achieve on your mat, but the physical and mental changes that it brings about and that you carry into your daily life.

MOST POWERFUL YOGA POSES

Other than when you are sleeping, you are either sitting or standing and often doing so for extended periods of time. While doing so, your body assumes its own habitual postural alignment, which may sometimes be good, sometimes so-so, and sometimes bad. Whatever the alignment happens to be, it feels normal because you are accustomed to it.

As stated throughout this book, practiced on a regular basis, yoga returns the body to balance and symmetry—stretching what is tight, strengthening what is weak, and returning range of motion to stiff joints. The frequency of your yoga practice determines how quickly these changes occur. Additionally, you can do many small yet powerful things on a daily basis that will aid this process. Some are mere reminders to give yourself a break from bad habits, and others are easy exercises to relieve overused and tired muscles. The most indispensable practice is also the simplest, because it can result in powerful changes: examining how you stand and sit.

Standing and Sitting

How do you stand when you are waiting for an elevator, in line at a store, or at a light waiting to cross the street? Do you stand on one leg, hip jutting to one side? Is your head down? Are your shoulders hunched and rounded? Are your feet turned outward? Do you stand the same way all the time, or do you shift from one pattern to another? Likewise, what are your habits when you sit, be it at a computer, at the dinner table, or on a sofa? Do you slouch into the back of the seat? Are your shoulders raised toward your ears? Is your upper back rounded? Is your head jutting forward? Take a moment to assess your habitual patterns, and do so several times throughout the day and over a period of time.

Equal standing and staff pose are two of the most powerful yoga poses. When you stand and sit this way, your weight-bearing joints are aligned: head over shoulders, shoulders over hips, hips over knees, and knees over ankles. The spine is aligned as nature intended, and so the weight on the lower back is neutralized. It is the most basic and yet most fundamentally essential alignment exercise to do on a daily basis.

There is no question that over time yoga will make you more aware of your harmful tendencies, and as your muscles gain balance in strength and flexibility, your body's natural alignment will change. To accelerate this process and gain instant benefits, you can make some simple modifications to how you stand, sit, and run. This takes your yoga practice off the mat and is one of the truly magical and powerful aspects of yoga.

Good posture is an essential component to running with ease and efficiency. Most (if not all) of us have brought our ingrained postural habits into running. For example, if your shoulders have been tight and hunched all day, they stay that way when you run. Furthermore, the effects of muscular imbalances are exacerbated by the weight-bearing impact of running. So, along with a regular yoga practice, changes in deeply rooted postural habits will make great strides in improving your running.

The following fundamental yoga poses have been modified to be done off the mat. A little goes a long way to breaking deeply engrained and detrimental patterns in your body. Accompanied with deep yogic breathing, you will energize your body, calm the mind, and be ready for the challenges that await.

Equal Standing

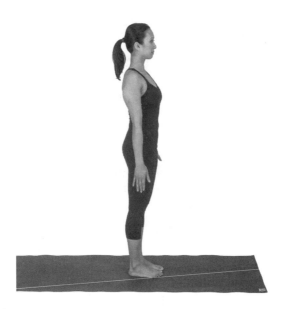

Description

1. See chapter 6 for a detailed description of this pose.

2. Remind yourself of this pose whenever you are standing. You can practice it regardless of your footwear. If you are wearing high-heeled shoes, be aware of the weight-shifting effect.

Key Points to Remember

- **Ground yourself.** Align the feet hip-distance apart so the toes are facing front. Press down evenly through the bases of the toes and heel.

- **Think tall.** Lengthen your spine as you draw the belly in and up.

- **Lengthen the neck.** Reach up through the crown of the head and align the head over the shoulders.

- **Open the chest.** Draw the upper arm bones back, press the shoulder blades down the back, and broaden through the chest.

Chair Staff Pose

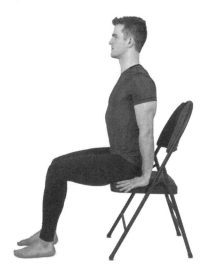

Description

1. See chapter 7 for a detailed description of staff pose. The alignment while seated in a chair is the same as staff pose, except that the legs are bent at 90 degrees.
2. Shift to the front of the seat so the back is not supported. The legs are bent at 90 degrees, with the knees over the ankles and the toes facing front.

Key Points to Remember

- **Sit upright.** Don't lean into the back of the chair. Sit forward on the chair and use the core muscles to support the torso.
- **Ground yourself.** Feel an even weight on both sitting bones.
- **Keep the legs symmetrical.** The legs are bent to 90 degrees, with the knees over the ankles. The feet and knees are hip-distance apart, with the toes facing front.
- **Keep the belly in.** Support the back by pulling in the front ribs and navel.
- **Open the chest.** Draw the upper arm bones back, press the shoulder blades down the back, and lift the breastbone.
- **Sit tall.** Lengthen the front, back, and sides of the body, and keep the head over the shoulders.

Computer Use

If you spend extended hours at a computer, some simple off-the-mat exercises can do wonders to relieve the aches and pains associated with repetitive strain. Do these often throughout the day. They take only a few moments of your time, and you will instantly reap the benefits.

In each pose, remember to take up to 5 deep, diaphragmatic breaths.

Spine

These simple variations of yoga poses rejuvenate and energize the spine and are super easy to do virtually anytime and anywhere. Through this simple series, you will stretch the spine to help decompress the lower back and increase blood flow to the spine. A simple spinal twist brings a healthy supply of blood to the back muscles and vertebrae while giving you an energy boost. A simple forward fold helps release tension in the back and shoulders and helps release physical and mental stress.

Desk Downward Dog

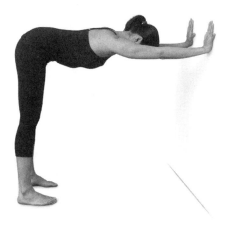

Description

1. See chapter 7 for a detailed description of downward dog.
2. In this variation, place the hands on the desk (or on a wall).

Key Points to Remember

- Press the hands firmly on the desk, shoulder-distance apart; walk the feet back until the arms straighten and the upper body is parallel to the floor.
- Strongly press the shoulder blades down the back. Keep the head in line with the shoulders.
- The feet are hip-distance apart, firmly and evenly grounded with the toes facing front.
- Position the hips over the knees, and keep the legs straight with quadriceps contracted. You may feel a stretch in the hamstrings as well as the spine.

Seated Chair Twist

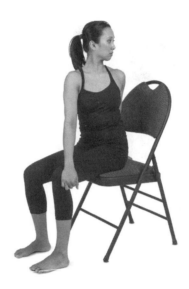

Description

1. Start in chair staff pose.
2. Place the left hand to either the back of the seat or arm of the chair, with the right hand at the outer left thigh.
3. Keeping the spine long and in alignment, twist to the left.
4. Hold, return to center, and repeat on the other side.

Key Points to Remember

- As you twist, ensure that the spine is upright and not leaning. Pull the navel in and contract both sides of the torso to deepen the twist.
- Keep the head aligned over the shoulders; do not let it drop or tilt.
- Keep the feet evenly and firmly grounded.

Chair Forward Bend

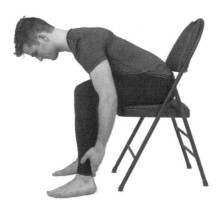

Description

1. Start in chair staff pose.
2. Lengthen the spine and fold forward, resting the chest on the thighs.
3. Let the hands slide down the shins and hold on to the ankles, or let them rest on the floor.
4. Keep extending the breastbone forward.
5. If unable to rest the chest on the thighs, extend forward and rest the head on the folded arms on the desk.

Key Points to Remember

- Do not round the back. Rather, lengthen the sides of the torso and slide the breastbone forward.
- Let the head be heavy, ensuring there is no strain at the front or back of the neck.

Neck and Shoulders

Many people suffer from chronic neck and shoulder tightness, and some quick stretching can bring instant relief. These exercises alleviate the buildup of tension in the neck and shoulders, help counteract the effects of shoulder hunching, and open the chest. Additionally, moving the shoulder joint through its range of motion reduces stiffness. All of the exercises in this section can be done while sitting or standing.

Simple Chest Stretch

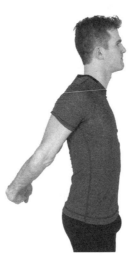

Description

1. This simple stretch can be done either sitting or standing.
2. Interlace the fingers behind the back. Roll the upper arm bones back, and draw the shoulder blades down the back. Do not pinch the shoulder blades together, rather firmly press them into the upper back.
3. Lift the breastbone, widen the collarbones, and press the hands toward the floor as you extend them away from the body.
4. Pull the front of the ribs in to engage the core.

Key Points to Remember

- Strongly press the shoulder blades into the body to fully open the chest.
- Breathe deeply to further expand the chest and energize the body and mind.

Cow Pose, Shoulder Stretch

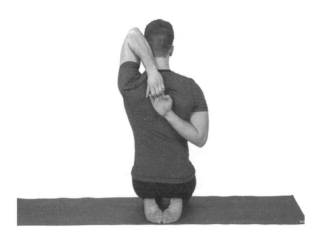

Description

1. See chapter 8 for a detailed description of this pose.
2. This pose can be done while standing or seated.
3. Do this several times throughout the day to improve the range of motion of the shoulder joints and release upper-back and shoulder tension.

Key Points to Remember

- Keep the shoulders pressed down.
- Imagine pulling the hands away from each other for a deeper stretch.

Ear to Shoulder

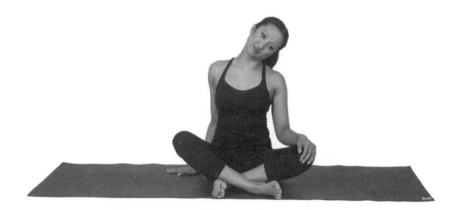

Description

1. See chapter 8 for a detailed description of this pose.
2. This pose can be done while seated on a chair.

Key Points to Remember

- Keep the spine straight. Ensure that the head is upright, in line with the spine, and not tilted to the side.
- Keep the shoulders down. Press the shoulder blades down the back, and let the weight of the head produce the stretch.

Hips

As detailed in chapter 10, the hip joints become locked in one position from sitting or standing for extended periods of time, leaving them tight and stagnant. This simple exercise can be done almost anywhere and encourages blood flow to the hip joints, reducing tightness and energizing and mobilizing this important part of the body.

Chair Hip Stretch

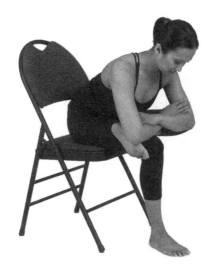

Description

1. To perform the exercise while standing, see knee to ankle balance pose (chapter 10).
2. To perform the exercise while sitting, start in chair staff pose. Place the left ankle on the right knee, flex the foot and actively press the thigh toward the floor, keeping weight even on the sitting bones. For a deeper stretch, fold forward with chest resting on folded leg.
3. Repeat on the other side.

Key Points to Remember

- Relax the muscles around the hip joint of the bent leg, and let the thigh fall heavily toward the floor. Do not press down on the knee of the bent leg.
- Relax the shoulders.

Wrists

Extended periods of time spent using computers also leads to tight wrists and forearms, which increases the risk of carpal tunnel syndrome. Simple actions such as making tight fists, rotating the wrists in both directions, and stretching and moving the fingers and wrists encourage blood flow to the hands and wrists. This tabletop stretch is intense but very effective to counteract the ill effects of overuse of computers.

Tabletop Wrist Stretch

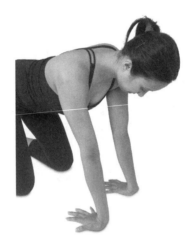

Description

1. Stand at the front of the desk. This stretch can also be done on the floor, as demonstrated.
2. Outwardly rotate the arms and hands so the fingers are facing toward you, and place them on the desk.
3. Position the hands beneath the shoulders and try to flatten the palms to the surface, with fingers spread and straight (as in downward dog).
4. Lean forward and press firmly into the palms and fingers.
5. Bend the elbows toward you.
6. Do this several times throughout the day.

Key Points to Remember

- This is less intense when you stretch one hand at a time.
- Ensure that the palms and fingers are spread and pressing down evenly.
- The bend in the elbow will be slight, but the effect is intense. With repetition, the bend will deepen and the discomfort will reduce.

Eyes

Sitting and staring at a computer screen for hours can cause eye strain and headaches. The muscles of the eyes also should be exercised to keep them healthy and toned. This simple exercise strengthens the muscles of the eyes and relieves eye soreness and strain; yet, at the same time, it energizes them.

Relieve Eye Strain

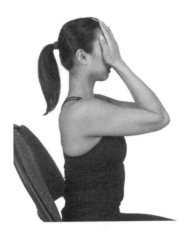

Description

1. Sit in chair staff pose.
2. Look away from the computer screen and focus your gaze outward at least 20 feet (6 m). Hold this gaze for at least 10 seconds.
3. Bring your gaze in closer to a midway point; hold this gaze for about 10 seconds.
4. Bring your gaze toward the tip of your nose and hold for about 10 seconds.
5. If your eyes are irritated, itchy, or dry, blink several times to moisten them.
6. Repeat the three-point gaze a number of times.
7. When you have completed the three-point gaze, rub the hands together to generate heat. Place the warm palms on the closed eyes and allow the heat to relax the eyes. Breathe deeply while doing this.

Key Points to Remember

- When shifting the gaze move the eyes slowly.
- Relax the forehead and keep the gaze soft.
- Do this several times throughout the day, particularly if you are spending extended periods of time at a computer.

Energize and Destress

Deep, diaphragmatic breathing is a simple way to energize the body. This is a simple tool that can be used anytime. When you are feeling tired or drowsy, when you are angry, when you feel overwhelmed or anxious, or when you are feeling stressed, take a few deep breaths. As few as five of these breaths will give you an instant energy boost and calm your body and mind as the added oxygen travels through your body and energizes every cell.

Deep Breathing

Description

1. See chapter 3 for a detailed description of ujjayi and abdominal breathing.
2. This can be done at any time, even while sitting at a computer. Concentrate on exhaling completely to empty the lungs, and then inhale to fill the lungs to capacity.
3. Try taking a few moments to perform this exercise prior to your run. Not only will this help establish a rhythm to your breathing that you can carry into your running, but it will also help you to clear your mind, sharpen your focus, and bring your mind and body into unison.

Key Points to Remember

- Breathe in and out through the nose.
- Focus on the sensation of filling the lungs and emptying them with every breath.
- As you breathe, focus on the sound and feel of the breath to keep the mind from wandering.

Chapter 14

Yoga and Injuries

By now you should be convinced that yoga is a perfect way to counterbalance the effects of running. A regular yoga practice will keep you on the road and, most important, make you a healthier runner. Through yoga, you will develop a deeper awareness and understanding of your body: your strengths, weaknesses, imbalances, and habitual tendencies. As you deepen your yoga practice, the patterns in your body will reveal themselves. One piece of information at a time, like a jigsaw puzzle, you will gain a better understanding of your body as a whole. You will learn to listen to the subtle messages your body continually communicates. Then it is up to you to decide what to do with that information.

Many runners keep running logs or journals, meticulously documenting their planned weekly runs. Depending on the training program, a rest day may be a day of no running, and a recovery day may include a short run. However, runners seldom include and document a yoga practice in their plans. Moreover, most runners are unlikely to include, or even consider, a yoga practice during a recovery phase. In many cases, yoga is what falls off the schedule because of time constraints.

Make room in your life for yoga. Build it into your training schedule by including it in your training log. When it is written down, it becomes more of a commitment, and you are less likely to put it off. Use your yoga practice to truly recover from draining runs. Don't be afraid to experiment with your training. Many runners have found that they can reduce their mileage, increase their yoga practice, and have the same or even better results on race day. This is because the body has maintained its capacity for running but is less physically exhausted.

Although a day off from running will rest your body, a yoga practice will provide the rest component while energizing and restoring the body and mind. Because yoga is the best vehicle for active recovery, let it become a lifelong companion to running. In return it will enable you to continue running for as long as you desire.

Maria's Story

I had run seven marathons and several half marathons before I realized that my body needed me to make time for yoga. My yoga practice started with one class a week. I felt great after each session and wanted more of this feeling. Soon I came to realize that once a week wasn't enough. I gradually increased my yoga practice to three times a week, and I found this to be a great balance with my running.

Yoga has helped me to pay more attention to my body and respond to the aches and pains caused by running sooner rather than ignore them and continue to push through discomfort or pain that often resulted in injury. In this way, yoga has helped me the most. Yoga has helped me to be more patient with my running and has allowed me to accept the new runner I am today. These days, I am very much at peace with my running and continue to feel free, energized, and strong on my runs. As long as I listen to my body, I can continue to run pain free and stay fit.

GOOD PAIN VERSUS BAD PAIN

Although yoga will certainly decrease your risk of injury, it is not a silver bullet, nor is it a guarantee that a running injury will not occur. With the exponential growth in yoga in recent years, much has been written about yoga injuries. Yoga is a physical practice, and as such it carries its own risk factors. So you may be thinking, "I am taking up yoga for its therapeutic benefits and to reduce my risk of injury. Now I face another type of risk?" Not to worry, because the benefits of yoga far outweigh the risks, and with proper attention to detail and a mindful practice, the risks can be mitigated. It is important to develop awareness, be present in mind and body during practice, and apply appropriate caution so that yoga serves your needs without harm.

On the surface, yoga may seem benign because it requires little movement. However, correct alignment is imperative to ensure that joints, ligaments, and tendons are protected at all times. A yoga practice needs to be approached with a respectful mind-set. Many poses require that you move your body and hold positions that may be completely foreign to you, especially if you are more adapted to quicker-moving athletic activities. This applies to the relatively simple poses, not to mention the pretzel-shaped poses commonly seen in the media. When you are stiff, stepping into a basic lunge can be a challenge, putting a strain on the hip flexors, hamstrings, or adductors.

Recall that yoga was not initially practiced for physical fitness. The purpose of the physical aspect was to prepare the body for meditation as a means of spiritual development and elevated consciousness. Yet the line between fitness and yoga has been blurred, and much has been written about seeking the yoga body. As yoga becomes more of an exercise system, large class sizes, loud music booming above the voice of the instructor, and quick-paced flows of postures can pose risks for the more inexperienced who are trying to keep up. Unfortunately, tight bodies that are in the greatest need of yoga also face the greatest risk in this type of environment. Understanding your body and where you are most at risk is crucial to developing a healthy and sustainable practice. In the end, you are primarily responsible for setting and maintaining your personal safety boundaries; do not be afraid to exit a situation that you deem dangerous.

As a runner, you may be accustomed to a no pain, no gain method of working out; if so, you will need to change your mind-set for yoga. Never aim to push to a point of pain in a yoga practice. That is not to say that you will not feel pain at times, but you need to become familiar with good pain versus bad pain. Most definitions of pain refer to an unpleasant sensation with degrees of intensity.

Those new to yoga commonly say they feel pain in poses that are challenging. When you feel pain during yoga, ask yourself whether it is a stretch pain or a sharp joint pain. Most commonly, it is from the stretch, yet it is important to know the difference. For example, stretching tight hamstrings typically registers as pain. However, if the source of the pain is in the belly of the muscle, it is good pain because it means that the muscle fibers are stretching. On the other hand, a sharp pain at the sitting bone is bad pain, because it means you are overstretching the hamstring tendon at its insertion point. By simply breathing through good pain, over time the intensity, or pain, will lessen. However, you need to avoid bad pain.

Over time and with proper guidance, you will be better able to differentiate the types of pain and use this information to define your personal limits. Knowing these limits and staying within them will help you develop an intelligent practice so you can gain the benefits of yoga without succumbing to a yoga injury.

YOGA SAFETY

The yoga sequences laid out in this book are designed specifically for runners. The details in each pose description ensure correct alignment when setting up in the poses. Then, as appropriate, we emphasize more specific muscle actions, often for stability. Take the time to read the full description, move into the pose slowly, and give yourself time to be in the pose, feeling the various sensations. If anything registers as pain, ensure that it is good pain. In this way you will gain the full benefit from each pose while avoiding the risk of injury.

Following are some safety guidelines to keep in mind as you enter or extend your yoga journey.

Build a Solid Foundation   You wouldn't think of running a marathon without doing the appropriate training, and you need to think similarly about yoga. It is best to start with a basic sequence and build to a more challenging one. A firm base of knowledge and some familiarity with the actions required in the poses will ensure a safe practice.

Take Your Time   Don't rush your practice. Take your time moving into the pose and adhere to the alignment principles. Always think of building your pose from the ground up, be it your feet, hands, or sitting bones. Then settle into the pose and breathe deeply. Don't be in a rush to come out of the pose, and when you do, remember that this is part of the pose also. If you are moving through a flow sequence, approach it the same way. At first, it may take you a bit longer to complete a sequence, but as your body gains mobility, you will move through poses with greater ease and efficiency.

Know Your Body   To do yoga safely and deepen your work without risk of injury, you need to know some anatomy. This is not to suggest that you bury your head in the *Gray's Anatomy* text. However, it is important to have an understanding of the basic skeletal structure and related muscles. For example, most runners know that their hamstrings are located along the backs of their upper thighs. But it is important to know where the tendon attachments are situated so that if a sharp sensation occurs at these points, the alarm sounds to back off. The more you know about your anatomy, the better equipped you will be to listen to the vital signals communicated either when running or practicing yoga. It is for this reason that some basic anatomy is included throughout the previous chapters. In addition, there are endless sources of anatomy information in print and digital formats. Make it a habit to peruse them from time to time and learn more about your makeup.

Listen to Your Body   Whether you are practicing yoga from this book, from a DVD, or in a class, you are your own teacher. One of the great gifts that yoga offers is getting to know your body and mind on a broader and deeper level. Do not underestimate the power of your own intuition or succumb to pressure to do something that doesn't feel right for your body. If you are experiencing pain and are not certain whether it falls in the category of good or bad pain, back off. It is better to play it safe. If any part of your body becomes numb, circulation is impaired. Come out of the pose, take a few deep breaths, and go back to the pose. If at any time you feel the need for a break, do not hesitate to move into a relaxing pose, but always stay with the yogic breathing.

Recognize Your Breathing Patterns   Aside from the physical sensations experienced in a yoga practice, your breath is a window to the internal environment. The pace, depth, and sound of your breath will let you know if you are overexerting. If at any time you find yourself gasping for air or short of breath, stop and move into a more relaxing pose. Focus on regaining an even diaphragmatic breathing pattern. As with running, the tougher the work, the more mindful you need to be of the breath; being in control of your breath is fundamental to both running and yoga.

Do Not Compete   Yoga is not a competitive sport, so leave your competitive tendencies for your races. If the person practicing beside you can flop into a forward bend with palms on the floor, don't feel you need to do so also. Similarly, if you see a picture of someone in a pose, don't form an image in your mind that drives you to mimic that pose. Always go back to the fundamentals of the pose and move into and through it mindfully with integrity, and respect your limits. This way you will stay within your own safety boundaries and gain the full benefits of the pose without the risk.

Find a Warm Space   Yoga is best done in a warm room, because the body is more limber when warm. You don't need extreme heat— just a room temperature that is comfortable when you are wearing a light layer of yoga attire. The purpose of the sun salutation done at the beginning of a yoga sequence is to create internal body heat. If you are doing one of the more challenging sequences, be prepared to sweat. When you are warm, you will go deeper into a pose, so don't try to push to the same point when you are cold.

MODIFYING YOUR YOGA PRACTICE

In spite of your best efforts, you may find yourself on your yoga mat with an injury, from running, yoga, or a run-of-the-mill mishap. Generally, runners are quite accustomed to dealing with running injuries and seek the treatment of a health professional, modify their training, or stop running for a period of time. Runners who experience a yoga injury sometimes draw the conclusion that yoga isn't for them and stop practicing. Dealing with a yoga injury may be less familiar and at times more frustrating than dealing with a running injury.

When a yoga injury occurs, there is always a solution. Most often the solution is yoga itself, but practiced in a different way. The injury most likely resulted from doing something incorrectly—repeated misalignment, overstretching, or being overly aggressive and pushing beyond a safety boundary. For the most part, if you have sustained a yoga injury, you can continue your yoga practice by adopting a different approach and perhaps modifying certain poses.

This section examines the most common types of yoga injuries and provides tips on how best to avoid them and, in the event of an injury, how to modify specific poses so that you can continue to practice. Try the simplest modification first, and if the problem persists, move to a deeper modification or stop doing the pose for a period of time. Just as in running, seek the advice and treatment of a professional health care provider when needed.

The injuries listed in table 14.1 are based on the yoga poses outlined in the sequences (chapter 12). All sequences in this book can be done with the type of injuries listed here by modifying them as noted. If needed, eliminate the troublesome poses from the sequence for a period of time. Modify your practice, but don't stop it.

You love to run . . . and hopefully, after some time, you will learn to love yoga also. Yoga has the unique capacity to improve your mental focus and your mental connection to your body, strengthen and tone your muscle mass, improve the range of motion in your joints, and improve your lung capacity. The benefits of yoga compound over time and, in addition to making you a healthier runner, will improve the quality of your daily life.

Despite its many benefits, yoga is a physical practice and should be approached and respected as such. Follow the alignment principles, but remember that every body is unique and that your uniqueness must be respected. Yoga poses and sequences can be modified to fit your body and physical state. The intensity of your yoga practice can be increased or decreased depending on your condition and energy level on a given day. Remember to include restorative poses when needed.

Table 14.1 Common Yoga Injuries and Suggested Pose Modifications

Body part	Source of pain	Correction	Modification(s)
Wrists	Bearing the body's weight on the hands in: Downward dog Plank Chaturanga Upward dog	Spread the fingers. Ground the base of the index fingers. Distribute weight through the entire palm. Contract the muscles of the arms and create a sensation of pulling the weight up through the arms and down the back. Press the hips back to reduce weight bearing in the upper body.	If pain is persistent and continues after practice, modify poses where pain is felt, and if needed, eliminate weight bearing for a time. Downward dog, plank—Do dolphin variation. Chaturanga—Avoid the pose. Upward dog—Do cobra variation.
Elbows	Weight bearing with straight arms in: Downward dog Plank Chaturanga Upward dog	Do not hyperextend the elbow joint. Contract the muscles of the upper arms and pull the shoulders down the back to reduce weight impact in the joints.	Downward dog, plank—Keep the inner elbows facing each other. Chaturanga—Keep the elbows in so they graze the upper body when lowering. Upward dog—Lift the chest and pull the shoulders down the back; keep a slight bend in the elbows.
Shoulders	All upper-body weight-bearing poses (often related to overuse)	Become familiar with the feeling of the shoulder blades moving down the back, away from the ears, and pressing into the upper ribs. Be mindful to find this action in all the poses, especially when weight bearing. Seek a balance of strength and flexibility in the shoulder joint. Strengthen weak upper-body muscles to support the shoulder joint, and balance with poses that stretch and increase range of motion. Avoid overextension of the shoulder joint. When the arms are extended, pull the arm bones into the sockets so they connect to the body.	It is best to find the appropriate shoulder action when there is no weight bearing, as in equal standing, equal standing with arms overhead, or downward dog at the wall. Duplicate this work in the poses that require greater weight bearing. Downward dog, plank—Pull the shoulder blades down the back to create space between the upper arms and the base of the neck. Chaturanga—Drop to the knees to reduce the weight and strain on the shoulders, or remain in plank and avoid the pose. Upward dog—Keep the shoulder blades pressing into the upper back both while in the pose, especially during the transition to upward dog. Regularly do the downward dog dolphin variation to build upper-body strength without compromising the shoulder joint. If needed, avoid weight-bearing poses for a period of time.

(continued)

Table 14.1 *(continued)*

Body part	Source of pain	Correction	Modification(s)
Neck	Tightening neck muscles Straining cervical vertebrae	In some poses it is appropriate to let the head be heavy and hang, such as in forward bends. However, this will feel right only when the forward bend deepens and the chest moves closer to the thighs. Until then, keep the head in line with the shoulders. Keep the head positioned in neutral over the shoulders in most poses.	Let the head drop heavily in downward dog. Find neutral spinal alignment in poses. Be mindful of the neck and avoid straining or tightening in all poses.
Lower back	Forward bending with rounded back Aggressive forward bending Spinal twists with spine misaligned Not engaging the core and letting the hips and belly sag in plank and chaturanga.	Pull the navel and lower ribs in to support the lower back. In forward bends, hinge forward from the hips and keep a neutral spine. If the back is rounded when seated, sit on a folded blanket for seated poses. In spinal twist poses, pull the belly in and lengthen the torso by lifting from the base of the spine. Strengthen the abdominals, especially the deeper transversus abdominis.	Bend the legs in forward bends. Ease up on the degree of forward bending. Avoid forward bends.
Knees	Misalignment in standing poses Hip-opening poses Hyperextension of the knee joint	Remember that the knee is a hinge, and avoid all torquing action. In all hip-opening poses, ensure that the external rotation is from the hip joint. Contract the quadriceps, especially the inner quads, to strengthen and support the knees. Do not hyperextend the knee joint. In standing poses, align the center of the knee with the center of the hip joint and the center of the ankle joint. In lunges, keep the front knee over the ankle joint. In seated poses, especially hip openers, ensure that the feet are flexed.	Ease off on seated hip-opener poses. In forward bending, keep the legs slightly bent. When seated in cross-legged poses, place a rolled blanket under the thighs. As long as there is no pain, regularly do the hero pose, supported as needed, and the wall squat.

Body part	Source of pain	Correction	Modification(s)
Ham-strings	Overstretching, primarily in standing forward bends Weak hamstrings	Ensure that the stretch is felt in the belly of the muscle with no sharpness at tendon insertion points. Contract the quadriceps in forward bends. Strengthen the hamstrings. Stretch the quadriceps.	Bend the legs. Ease up on the depth of forward bends. Avoid standing forward bends. Do only eccentric hamstring stretches.

Throughout your yoga journey, be mindful of your personal boundaries. That is, find your edge . . . but do not go over it! Listen to the inner voice that guides you. There is nowhere to get to in a yoga practice. As the yoga guru Geeta Iyengar eloquently summarized: "Yoga has a beginning, but has no end."

About the Author

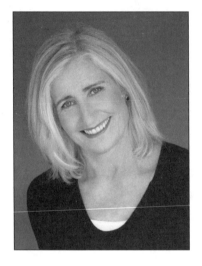

With an extensive history as a long-distance runner and yoga instructor, **Christine Felstead** has married her twin passions into a pioneering program for runners. She teaches yoga classes and workshops for runners and endurance athletes. Her *Yoga for Runners* teacher training program offers certification to a growing number of instructors now working in the United States, Canada, Mexico, and the United Kingdom. Felstead presents regularly at International Yoga Expos and canfitpro conferences and has produced two best-selling DVDs on yoga for runners. For additional information, visit www.yogaforrunners.com. She has been featured in numerous publications, including *Runner's World*, *Women's Running*, *Yoga Journal*, *Women's Health*, *Library Journal*, and Canada's *National Post*. She resides in Toronto.